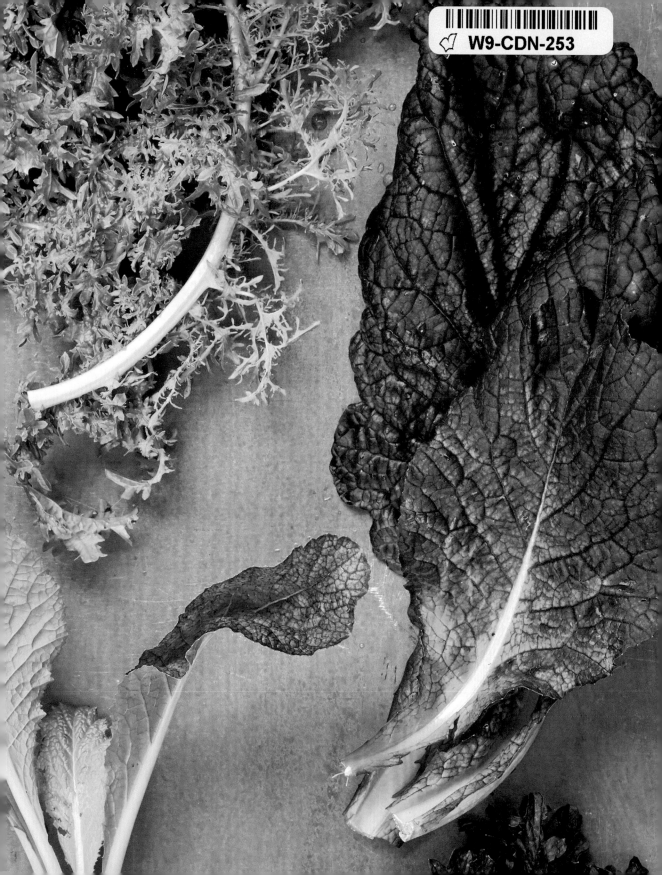

By

DANA JACOBI

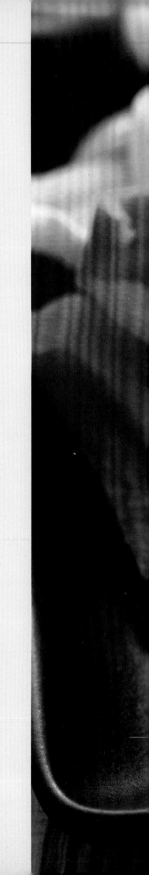

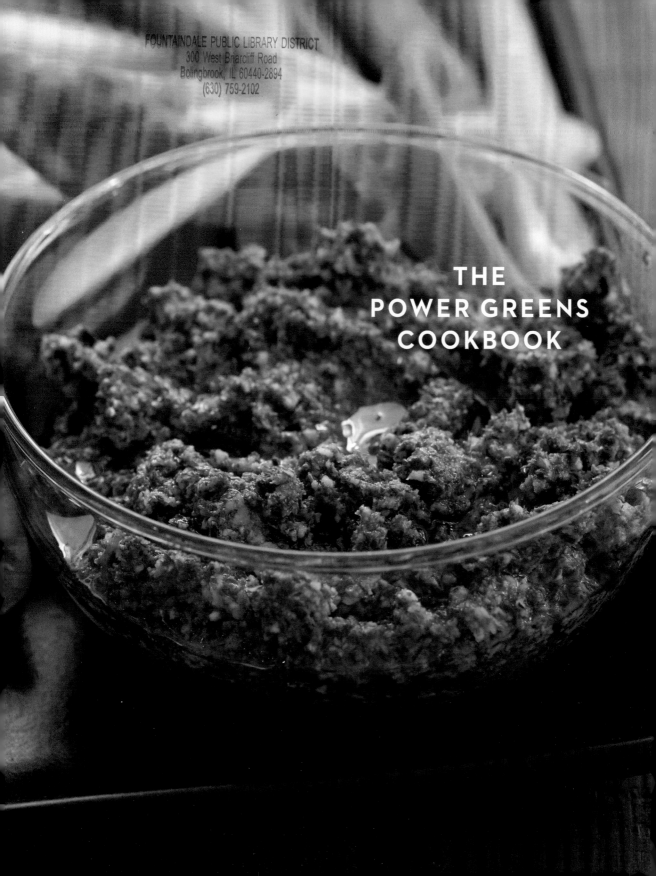

THE
POWER GREENS
COOKBOOK

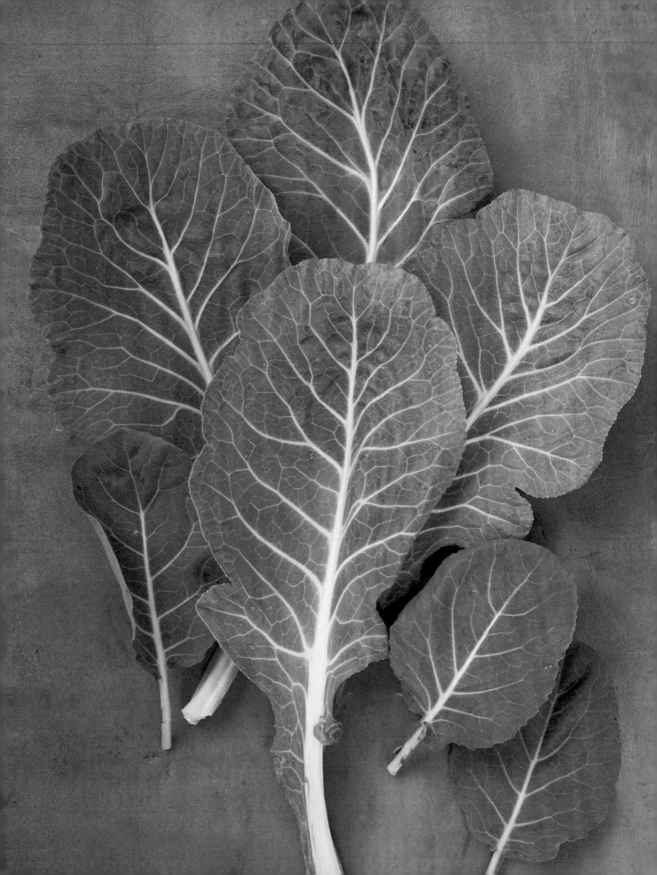

THE POWER GREENS

COOKBOOK

140 DELICIOUS SUPERFOOD RECIPES

DANA JACOBI

BALLANTINE BOOKS | NEW YORK

A Ballantine Books Trade Paperback Original

Copyright © 2015 by Dana Jacobi

All rights reserved.

Published in the United States by Ballantine Books, an imprint of Random House, a division of Penguin Random House LLC, New York.

BALLANTINE and the HOUSE colophon are registered trademarks of Penguin Random House LLC.

Photography by Ben Fink

LIBRARY OF CONGRESS CATALOGING-IN-PUBLICATION DATA
Names: Jacobi, Dana, author.
Title: The power greens cookbook : 140 delicious superfood recipes / Dana Jacobi.
Description: New York : Ballantine Books, [2015] | Includes index.
Identifiers: LCCN 2015037998 | ISBN 9780553394849 (pbk. : alk. paper) | ISBN 9780553393088 (ebook) Subjects: LCSH: Cooking (Vegetables) | Pasta salads. | Salads. | Soups. | Functional foods. | LCGFT: Cookbooks.
Classification: LCC TX801 .J333 2015 | DDC 641.6/5—dc23
LC record available at http://lccn.loc.gov/2015037998

Printed in China on acid-free paper

randomhousebooks.com

2 4 6 8 9 7 5 3 1

Book design by Barbara M. Bachman

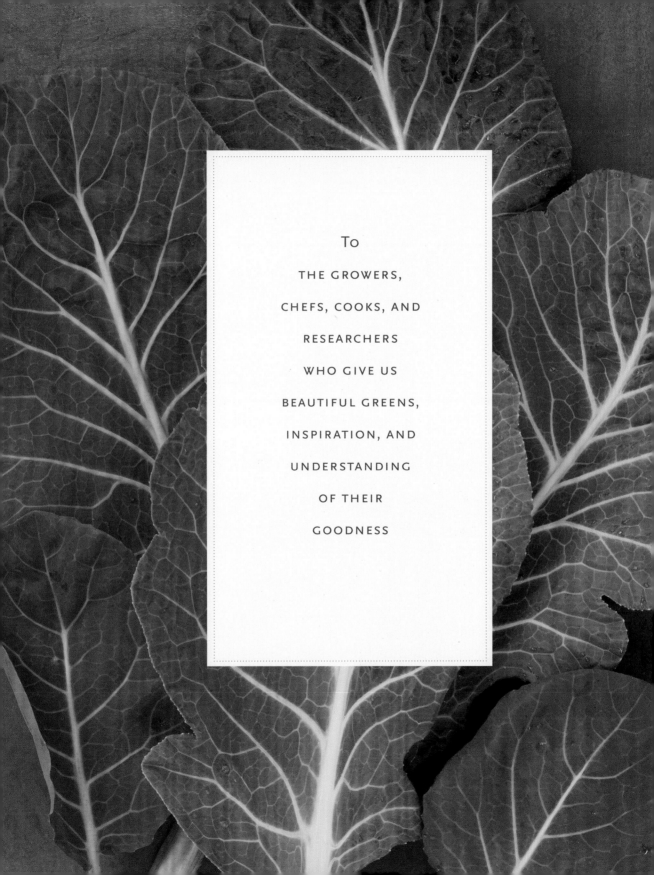

To

THE GROWERS,

CHEFS, COOKS, AND

RESEARCHERS

WHO GIVE US

BEAUTIFUL GREENS,

INSPIRATION, AND

UNDERSTANDING

OF THEIR

GOODNESS

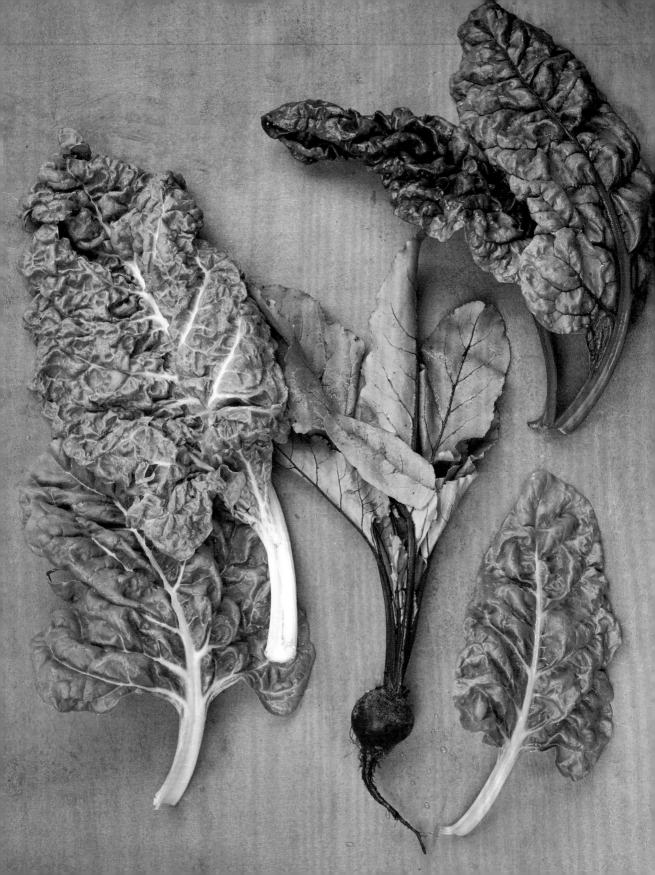

FOREWORD

AS A DIETITIAN WHO HAS WORKED WITH PATIENTS FOR OVER A DECADE TO use food to improve and maintain their health, too often I hear patients say they are either intimidated or frustrated by greens. They say, "I know I should eat (more) greens but I don't know how to cook them so that they will taste good." It is not just knowledge of the health benefits of greens that provides power. We need to know how to prepare them easily and make them taste so great that we get excited enough to buy them and prepare them. Thus, it is the combined knowledge of the health power of greens and easy great-tasting ways to prepare them that provides true power. So that's why I am thrilled that one of my favorite cookbook authors, Dana Jacobi, created this book that does both, beautifully and simply.

A word about health: These fifteen leafy dark greens deliver nutrients that will actually improve the health of every part of your body. At your core, greens improve digestion by helping to remove toxins from the body as well as helping promote a healthy pH level that in turn creates a more suitable environment for good bacteria (probiotics). As we age, our bodies need nutrient support to protect all our cells and maintain the health of organs large (skin) and small (eyes). Dark greens do all of this, especially because of their high concentration of certain nutrients. Leafy Power Greens are one of the most important sources of different antioxidants—vitamins and minerals as well as plant nutrients (phytonutrients). These antioxidants play a critical role as our body's cleanup team. They seek out the "dirt" (free radicals) that life's stresses, food, environmental toxins, and the general workload in the body produce. Thus, consuming Power Greens regularly helps maintain a clean, healthy body from the inside out.

A word about taste: From our first bite, taste dictates whether or not we like something, and very few people will continue to eat foods they don't like, even if they know how good they are for them. Over the years, I have counseled plenty of clients who suffer through eating foods that they don't like the taste of by rewarding themselves with foods and beverages that they do find tasty or by making every effort to disguise or alter the taste of the food ingredient they dislike. Unfortunately, these efforts haven't helped them get healthier; in fact, typically it's the opposite. I don't believe we should ever eat something we don't like the taste of in the name of enabling health. So the key is to learn to make healthy food taste great, and to have choices, as we all aren't going to like the same foods as others, nor will we necessarily like the same foods throughout our own life stages.

A word about quality: As a Qualitarian (someone who knows that better quality choices enable better health), I would be remiss to not say a word about the role of quality in the health power of foods, especially greens. The power of the dark, leafy greens described in this book comes from both what they contain and what they don't have on or in them. Many greens are on the Environmental Working Group's Dirty Dozen list, which means that their levels of pesticides tested among the highest in produce. That means that bite for bite and sip for sip they could contain greater amounts of pesticides than other produce, unless grown according to organic practices. That's not a reason to skip greens, but it's certainly a reason to choose organic greens as a way to reduce exposure to pesticides. After all, if a reason to eat Power Greens is to get their cleanup power, why would we eat greens with added toxins sprayed on them or on the soil in which they grow? That's like wearing dirty shoes while mopping the floor! So make an effort to buy organic produce grown with fewer or no pesticides. Purchasing organic can seem to present challenges from availability to cost, so it's good to know that many organic greens today cost close to or the same as chemically farmed versions. Additionally, one can save money and have year-round access by purchasing frozen organic (just as acceptable as "ready to eat"), which also prevents spoilage concerns.

A word on variety: Our minds and bodies benefit from variety in all, and our greens are no exception. Variety in taste, appearance, and preparation methods contributes to the absolute power of these fifteen greens. So challenge yourself to read about and try the greens you haven't eaten or don't normally have to eat. And if you already consume a green mentioned here, try out a new way to prepare it. What's interesting about greens, and all vegetables really, is that the different preparation methods actually promote different nutrients and amounts absorbed as well as giving you additional nutrients from the other ingredients in a recipe. So as you consider your weekly meal plans, decide what to bring to a party or a work potluck, or seek choices to improve your health, make sure to check out the awesome power of the fifteen powerful dark, leafy greens and recipes in this cookbook. I know I can't wait to dig into them!

—Ashley Koff, R.D.
ashleykoffapproved.com

CONTENTS

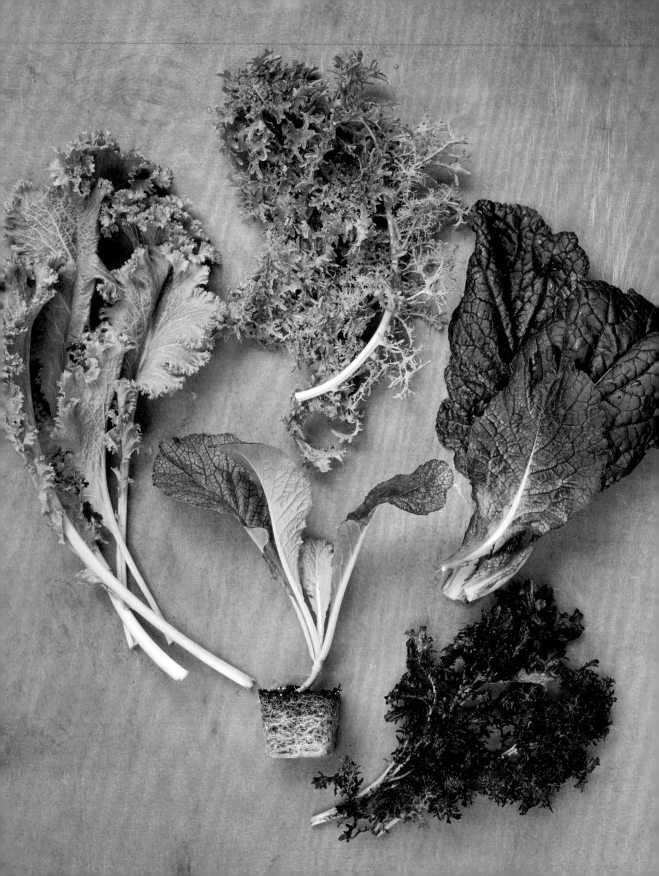

INTRODUCTION

WHETHER YOU LOVE DARK, LEAFY GREENS OR EAT THEM RELUCTANTLY, THIS book is for you. For greens lovers, here are recipes to enlarge your cooking repertoire plus new, useful preparation techniques. For everyone, here are delicious ways to work with the assertive flavors of the most nutritionally powerful leafy greens and ways to combine them with other healthy ingredients for mouthwatering results.

Shoppers I chat with at the market and students in my cooking classes ask the same questions: What to look for in greens and what to do with them? They first want to know how to buy the best greens; then they want to learn enticing ways to prepare them, not just for every day but also for special occasions.

I was lucky because my mother was a foodie and a health nut, a good cook and a great teacher. I grew up eating gourmet salads spiked with watercress, green cabbage topped with melted cheese, and fresh kale sautéed in butter. (Back then butter was considered the healthy fat.) I was in my twenties before I realized that my love of kale, cabbage, and other strong-tasting greens was unusual.

Every week, my mother taught me something new about buying and preparing foods. I learned to pick out beets with nice greens to steam. She showed me how to choose a good head of romaine lettuce because iceberg was "empty food." From Chinatown, we brought home greens we did not even have names for. An Italian neighbor showed us how to cook the broccoli rabe grown in her brother's garden. Most of all, Mom taught me to be adventurous, to try new foods, and to be fearless in the kitchen.

I want to inspire in you the same adventurous spirit by sharing recipes that make eating these dark, leafy greens irresistible. I will also walk you through buying each of them, explain the best way to keep them at home and how to prep them. You will learn the basic way to prepare each of these greens and find ways that fit them into your everyday eating without using a recipe. So think of this as more than a cookbook. Use it as a manual for shopping, storing, and enjoying fifteen potent greens packed with vitamins, minerals, and other health-promoting substances that can even help save your life.

I wrote *The Power Greens Cookbook* so you can eat these delicious dark greens every day and look forward to it. Through innovative recipes, I aim to make you comfortable buying and using so many kinds of greens that you truly enjoy greening your plate.

LEGEND FOR RECIPES

These symbols will help you find the dishes that fit your dietary and time needs.

(VG)   Vegetarian dish

(V)   Vegan dish or where vegan option is given

(GF)   Gluten-free dish

(30)   Dish ready in 30 minutes or less

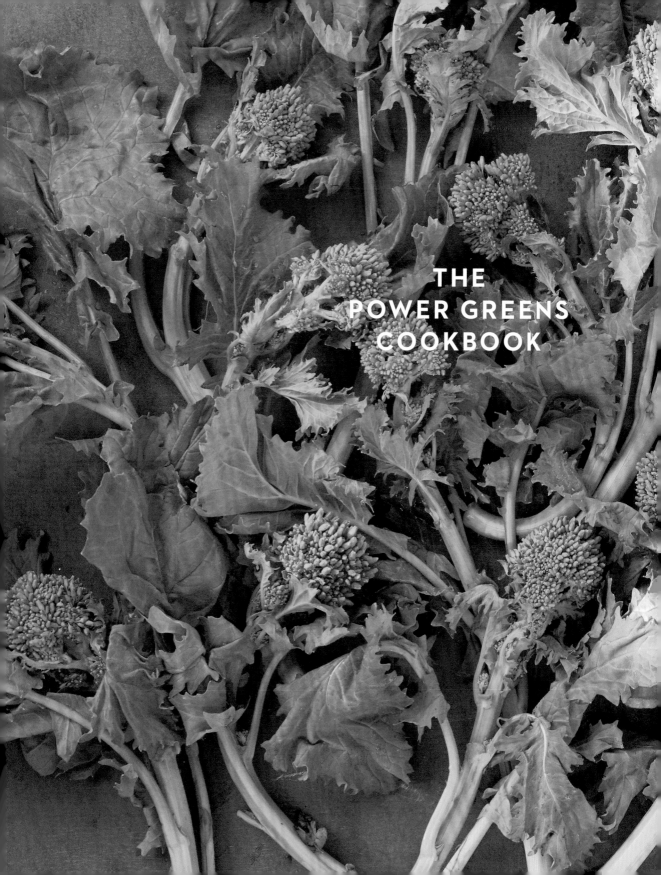

THE
POWER GREENS
COOKBOOK

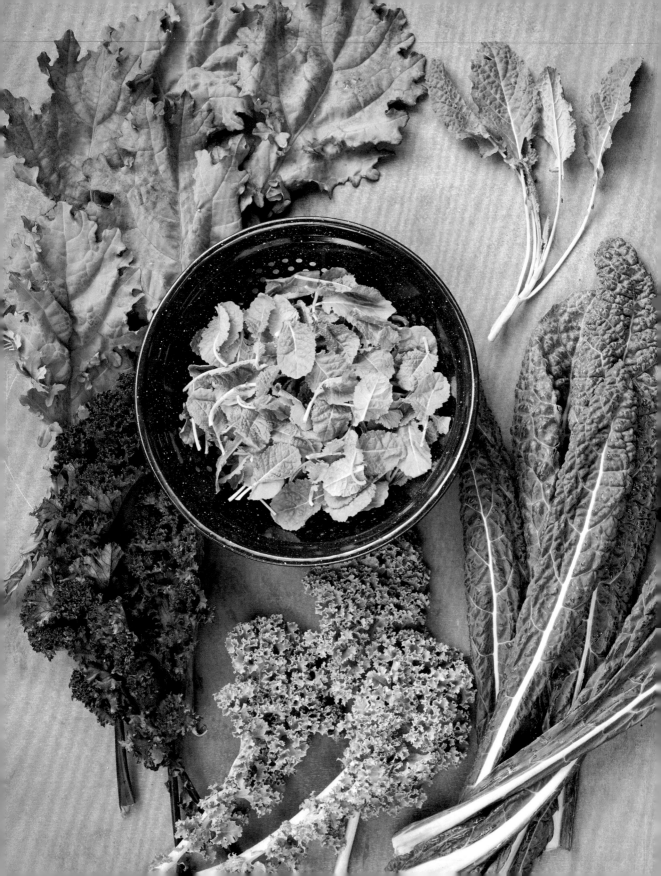

1.
THE POWER of GREENS

THE BENEFITS FROM EATING POWER GREENS ARE VAST— ranging from maintaining strong bones to protecting against cancer from head to toe, inside and out, including warding off skin cancers. They contain substances that neutralize and help eliminate toxins that accumulate in our bodies. Eating them helps reduce the risk of diabetes and strokes. Including them in your diet keeps your mind keen and your vision sharp.

These fifteen dark, leafy greens are dense with health-supporting nutrients and phytochemicals that protect against heart disease and high blood pressure and neutralize free radicals caused by inflammation and aging. No wonder we keep hearing more reasons why they belong in our diet every day. To put it bluntly, eating Power Greens can save your life.

Along with a wealth of vitamins, minerals, and unique phytonutrients, many of these greens contain as much fiber as a bowl of oatmeal, or even more. Some also contain a useful amount of protein, which is particularly helpful in a meatless diet. All this goodness makes them powerful indeed.

THE FIFTEEN POWER GREENS

These fifteen dark, leafy greens stand above other vegetables
because of substances found in each of them—often in high
concentrations—and what these do for our bodies. All vegetables
have nutritional benefits, but these in particular stand
head and shoulders above the rest.

ARUGULA

BOK CHOY

BROCCOLI LEAF

BROCCOLI RABE

BRUSSELS SPROUTS

CABBAGE

CHARD AND BEET GREENS

CILANTRO

COLLARD GREENS

KALE

MUSTARD GREENS

PARSLEY

ROMAINE LETTUCE

SPINACH

WATERCRESS

. . .

What Is in Them?

Some of the substances in these greens are familiar vitamins and minerals. Spinach contains lavish amounts of folate and iron. Collard greens provide a hefty amount of calcium, a mineral important for everyone but especially for vegans and others who do not eat dairy foods. Many of the top greens are excellent sources of vitamin K, which scientists are learning has more and more important functions than previously realized.

In addition to these valuable vitamins and minerals, most of these greens are rich in carotenoids, a family of antioxidants. These carotenoids include lutein and zeaxanthin, which protect our eyes against macular degeneration.

Less familiar phytonutrients abound as well in these greens. Glucosinolates, indoles, sulfuraphane, and antioxidant flavonoids are powerful enough to detoxify harmful substances that come from the environment and from foods we consume. They eliminate cancer-causing toxins, protect the heart and vascular system, and reduce the DNA damage free radicals cause.

There are fifteen of these Power Greens (actually nineteen if you count red and Napa cabbages, beet greens, which are close to chard, and both broccoli leaf and an heirloom broccoli in leaf form). Each of them, with its beneficial nutrients, is described in detail in its individual section after the recipes.

Why So Many Brassicas

Ten Power Greens are brassicas, aka cruciferous vegetables. Crucifers are a varied and supercharged botanical family. The ones included here—some darker, others more leafy—are arugula, bok choy, broccoli rabe, Brussels sprouts, cabbages, collard greens, kale, broccoli leaf, mustard greens, and watercress. Like other crucifers, such as radishes and broccoli, these greens taste hot or bitter because of the abundance of sulfur compounds and other phytochemicals they contain. For the plant, these substances provide protection. For us, they act as detoxifiers and often have anticancer properties, along with many other benefits, as explained in the section for each vegetable.

Substances in cruciferous vegetables called isothiocyanates are known as goitrogens because they have the potential to affect thyroid function. No carefully conducted studies have determined a relationship between them and changes in thyroid function for healthy individuals. I have a thyroid condition called Hashimoto's disease, and my endocrinologist, an eminent expert, assures me that eating generous amounts of kale, collards, and other brassicas has not caused or affected this. Cooking reduces the amount of these heat-sensitive goitrogens. Eating up to two to three cups a week of cruciferous vegetables is generally considered fine, but check with a healthcare professional if you are concerned about the goitrogens in brassicas, which include radishes, turnips, and other vegetables as well as broccoli and other dark greens.

Other Greens Excel, Too

Spinach, chard, and beet greens contain an abundance of folate and other vitamins and iron and other minerals. They are also extremely rich in carotenoids, which you want to make your skin look good and to protect against various cancers.

Lettuce does not top the list for nutrient density, but the B vitamins in romaine, plus its amounts of vitamins C and K, qualify romaine as a Power Green, especially its dark outer leaves. So one of my missions is showing you ways to love these greener, stronger-tasting leaves.

Two Herbs Are Tops

Parsley and cilantro come next. These fresh herbs are so rich in phytonutrients, vitamins, and carotenoids that I recommend eating them as abundantly as vegetables. Recipes here use them often—cumulative amounts count—and show how to enjoy them in larger amounts than usual.

LET'S BE REAL

If you don't like a food, or if preparing it takes too long, you won't bother with it. Four issues, I find, affect how willing people are to prepare and eat the most nutrient-powerful greens.

Taste

The good stuff in these greens is bitter by nature. What makes them so beneficial simply does taste bitter or pungently hot—or both, in the case of arugula, mustard greens, and watercress. As humans, we are biologically wired to like sweetness. And while other cultures accept and even embrace bitter foods, Americans remain notoriously averse to bitterness.

Texture

Dark greens are tough customers. Even romaine takes more chewing than other lettuces. But rather than making kale, collards, chard, and other greens pleasantly tender, many recipes undercook them, leaving them too chewy and pungent or tannic tasting.

Time

Many of these greens are high maintenance to prepare. Using kale, collards, leafy broccoli, chard, and mustard greens requires stripping out their tough stems and center vein one leaf at a time. Sometimes two-step cooking makes them more enjoyable.

Technique

The fourth resistance I hear about dark, leafy greens is not knowing what to do with many of them. This includes being unsure how much to buy and how to store them.

A SIMPLE SOLUTION

Two cooking techniques solve issues about cooking kale, collards, and other greens.

> Short Cooking: Plunging them briefly into one or two inches of boiling water

> Quick Cooling: Swiftly chilling Short Cooked greens under cold running water

Together, these techniques speed up blanching, then shocking dark greens. They reduce bitterness yet keep vivid taste.

Short Cooked–Quick Cooled greens used in dishes actually reduce their total cooking times. From start to finish, braised Tuscan kale is tender and ready in twenty rather than forty minutes. And it tastes better.

You can refrigerate the lightly cooked greens for up to three days, letting you prep several kinds efficiently on a weekend or during an evening, then use them during the week. They are ready to freeze, too.

Dishes made with greens that are Short Cooked and Quick Cooled have better texture. Some people are fine eating kale cooked for only five minutes, until just beyond collapsing, but don't be surprised if your jaw aches after chewing a few forkfuls. I like kale to have body, and broccoli rabe to be al dente, but not so much that eating them feels like work. I don't want my Brussels sprouts to bite back. Using these two steps gives you greens with the right texture to complete dishes more quickly and with the best flavor.

As if all this isn't enough, there is one more benefit to Short Cooking and Quick Cooling greens. Chard, beet greens, and collard greens release dark juices that turn soups and stews an unappealing color. Short Cooking before you use them in a recipe eliminates this problem.

HOW TO SHORT COOK–QUICK COOL GREENS

Boil 4 to 8 cups of water in a large saucepan. Add fresh greens and use a wooden spoon to push them until they collapse into the water. Cover and cook the greens for 2 to 4 minutes. Drain the greens in a colander and swish them under cold running water to chill them, which takes 30 seconds.

For buying greens, the first question I am asked is how to select them. The individual section on each Power Green at the back of the book gives a detailed description of what you want. It includes what to look for at your supermarket and local farmer's markets.

How much do I need to buy is usually the next question. Most of the Power Greens are sold in bunches. So how many bunches do you need?

HOW BIG IS A BUNCH?

Power Greens sold in a bag or plastic box contain a fixed weight, which makes buying the right amount easy. The Nutrition Facts labels show how many servings they provide. But there is no consistent answer for bunches because they have no fixed weight or size. More precisely, what a bunch weighs or contains is up to the farmer or grower. It is what he or she feels is right for kale, collards, broccoli leaf, arugula, parsley, and other greens. For spinach or watercress, the amount the person picking it can grasp and band determines the size of a bunch.

This vague measurement challenges cooks. But how vague is it? Using the scale every produce department has for customer use, I have weighed scores of bunches and found that for each green, there is a predictable range and an average weight. The recipes here use these as a guideline. If you, too, weigh bunches for a few weeks, your eye will get to recognize pretty closely what they weigh. Happily, most of the recipes here are flexible, so if you have a few more ounces of raw greens than called for, combine the extra with other greens in another dish, freeze them, or juice them.

BE PICKY

At the store, inspect both bags and boxes—including the bottom—to make sure the contents are all in good condition.

When you get home, dump the contents into a large bowl and pick through them for crushed, spoiled leaves. Also discard pieces of tough stem, which will stay hard and tough when cooked. Cut off dry, browned ends of packaged Brussels sprouts, broccoli rabe, or watercress.

> **Always** *wash packaged greens. Even immaculate-looking ones labeled triple-washed can have undesirable bacteria clinging to them.*

FROZEN GREENS

Commercially frozen greens save time, but spinach is the only one I recommend. Commercially frozen kale, collards, broccoli rabe, and Brussels sprouts taste watery. During cooking they can go quickly from tough or stringy to mushy. But I encourage freezing greens at home. A time-saver at mealtime, home-frozen kale, collards, broccoli leaf, and broccoli rabe are actually more tender when defrosted. You can braise them or use them in pasta dishes, soups, and stews with excellent, flavorful results.

Home-frozen spinach is also excellent.

STRIPPING

I remove the stem and center vein from the large-leafed Power Greens. For Tuscan kale, this includes taking out even the thin part near the top of the leaf. For collard greens and chard, the even texture when they are cooked without their central vein is infinitely nicer.

With slight practice, I promise you will strip the average bunch of greens in two minutes. There are two ways to do it.

Fold and Tear Hold a leaf in one hand, stem pointing up. With your other hand, bring the two dark, front sides of the leaf toward each other, like closing a book. Placing one hand at the base of the leaf, with your other hand pull the leaf out and away from the vein. To keep a firm grip, move your hands down the vein as the leaf tears away.

This works best with kales, broccoli leaves, mustard greens, beet greens, and smaller chard and collard greens.

V-Cut Lay a leaf flat on a cutting board, right side up and with the stem toward you. Starting at the top of the center vein, run the knife down along each side. Lift out and discard the vein and stem.

This is the best way to strip large leaves of chard, collards, and cabbage.

WASHING AND STORING

Wait until you're ready to use greens before washing them. They last longer this way, even if they are gritty or dirt is clinging to stems or roots.

Wash greens in a big bowl, not the sink. This avoids possible contamination. Getting most greens clean requires several water changes, so using a bowl requires less water. It lets you see better, too, when the water is clear and you are done.

My preferred way to store greens is to loosely wrap them in a paper towel, then slip them inside a plastic bag, stems facing the opening. Leave the bag open or close it loosely. Every couple of days, check and change the towel. Turn the bag inside out if too much moisture has collected inside it.

The section about each Power Green at the back of the book has more specific, individual storage instructions.

THE BIG SQUEEZE

Defrosted spinach and Short Cooked greens are full of water. To eliminate it, gather up the hardier greens and press them into a big ball. If your hands are small, like mine, make two balls.

For the softer greens—broccoli rabe, chard, and spinach—squeeze them out a handful at a time. Compress the handful in your fist until it is a firm roll; you don't have to wring it out like laundry. Then put a couple of the rolls together and squeeze them again.

HOW MUCH IS A CUP?

For a loosely packed cup, fill a dry measuring cup (see Good Technique) to the top with greens. For packed or firmly packed, keep adding to the full cup, pressing gently on the greens for packed, and pressing harder for firmly packed.

EQUIPMENT

These six tools will help you prep and cook Power Greens efficiently.

Scale: You should have one anyway, but for greens, use it to weigh bunches and loose leaves. My digital scale gives weights in ounces and pounds or in grams, which is useful for baking.

Large Saucepan with a Cover: A lightweight and non-reactive pot is helpful for Short Cooking greens. I use an All-Clad 4-quart stainless steel pot. It is big enough to Short Cook up to 2 pounds of stripped collard leaves or three 8-ounce bunches of spinach. A bigger pot is fine, but this size is easy to handle. The tighter the cover fits, the better.

Tongs: Use them to lift greens out of pots and to turn and move greens while sautéing them or when making kale chips. My favorite tongs, made of inexpensive metal, are 9 inches long, which gives more control than longer ones.

Spider or Skimmer: Chefs use this shallow metal basket on the end of a long handle to lift foods from liquid. A skimmer with a 5-inch basket or larger is useful for collecting greens when you Short Cook them. Use one that is pierced or has wires spaced close together, not the Asian-style basket made of widely spaced chicken wire that allows chopped greens to fall through.

Colander: Needed for draining greens and then cooling them under cold running water. Avoid aluminum—it can affect the taste of some greens when they are hot.

Large Bowl: For washing greens, I use a 4-quart bowl.

Since I cook one or more Power Greens every day, I store the colander, skimmer, and tongs together in the bowl so they are quickly at hand.

KNOWLEDGE IS POWER

This information will help you understand why Power Greens require the handling they do.

It's Alive After they are picked, greens are still alive and breathing. The faster they respire, the faster greens wilt and turn yellow. The colder they are kept, the more slowly they respire, which helps them stay vital longer.

Alive Means Vulnerable Sturdy as they look, many Power Greens wilt quickly when not kept cold. Get them home and into the fridge as quickly as possible and keep them well chilled. Plus when I set my refrigerator below 38 degrees, the shelf life of greens and everything else in it improves noticeably.

Alive Means Active As greens breathe, they exhale gases and lose moisture. This water collects inside a plastic bag holding lettuce or other leafy greens. The colder greens are, the more slowly they breathe and the longer they last. Watch for condensation inside the plastic bag, which encourages spoilage. To remove it, turn the bag inside out, first giving it a good shake. If the paper towel wrapping the greens is more than lightly moist, change it. Then slip the greens back into the bag, leaving it loosely closed so gases can escape and the greens can stay crisp and keep their color longer.

Alive Means Variable Arugula or collard greens picked from a field in May taste different from those harvested in August from the same field because the hot summer sun makes them tougher and more pungent. Spinach locally grown may be available only in spring and after summer's heat passes because it bolts in hot weather. Minerals and the amount of moisture in the soil affect the taste of greens, too. These are more reasons to be Zen about greens, preparing them based on what you have.

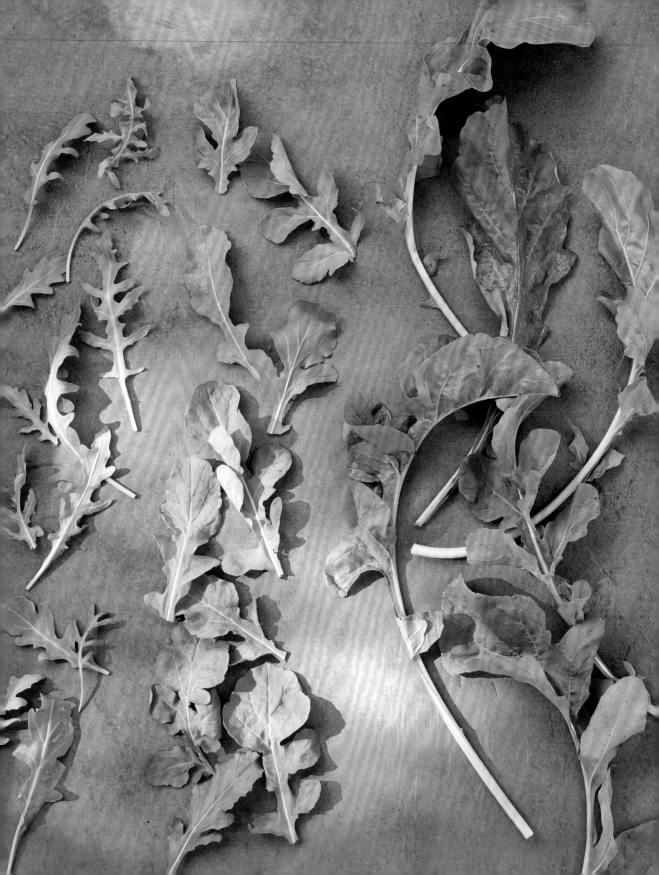

2.

DIPS, SPREADS, and BITES

THESE ARE DISHES I SERVE TO FAMILY AND GUESTS BEFORE a meal, just to take the edge off appetites while waiting to sit down at the table. There is also fuller fare I set out when I suspect lingering over drinks means that these nibbles and hors d'oeuvres may become our meal. They all go with alcohol—wine, beer, or cocktails—and with iced tea or mocktails. Many, like White Bean and Broccoli Rabe Bruschetta (p. 18), Brussels Sprouts Pinzimonio (p. 15), Kale Pesto with Carrot and Sweet Pepper Crudités (p. 21), and Roasted Red Peppers Stuffed with Kale (p. 31), are Mediterranean in flavor. Assembling several of them together makes a fine antipasto. Add a cheese board and you have a casual spread perfect for grazing. You can also pack Watercress Deviled Eggs (p. 22) for a picnic, enjoy Shrimp with Green Herb Mayonnaise (p. 28) while hanging out on the deck, or let sports fans dig into Mexican Seven Layer Dip (p. 25) and Hummus with Arugula and Parsley (p. 24) in front of the TV.

With choices for vegetarians, vegans, and carnivores, these dishes use eleven kinds of greens in all. All of the ingredients here are delicious as well as rich in health benefits.

BRUSSELS SPROUTS PINZIMONIO

SERVES 6 TO 8 |

In Italy, raw vegetables served with seasoned olive oil as a dip are called pinzimonio. Here, I dip lightly steamed Brussels sprouts into salsa verde, garlic-and-herb-infused olive oil made more piquant by mustard and capers. Also serve the sauced Brussels sprouts as a side dish with salmon, roast chicken, or sliced flank steak.

SALSA VERDE

2 teaspoons capers, preferably salt-cured

1 large garlic clove

1 medium shallot, coarsely chopped

½ lightly packed cup flat-leaf parsley

1 teaspoon Dijon mustard

1 teaspoon white wine vinegar

⅓ cup extra-virgin olive oil, preferably a grassy and pungent one, such as Sicilian Olio Verde

Salt and freshly ground pepper

. . . . . .

1 pound Brussels sprouts, small to medium size

CAPERS, SALT-CURED VERSUS PICKLED

Capers preserved in salt deliver more of their unique flavor than the vinegar-preserved kind. Before soaking, brush off the sea salt clinging to them and save it to use in tomato sauce or tuna salad.

---

1. Soak the salt-cured capers in ½ cup of water for 20 minutes. Drain and rinse the capers in a strainer under cold water. For vinegar-soaked capers, rinse and drain. Set the capers aside.

2. In a mini food processor, pulse the garlic, shallot, and parsley until the parsley is coarsely chopped, 10 to 12 pulses. Add the mustard, vinegar, and capers and pulse until the parsley is finely chopped. Transfer the parsley mixture to a small bowl, whisk in the oil, and season with salt and pepper to taste. Set the sauce aside for 20 minutes to let the flavors develop.

3. While the sauce sits, trim the stems from the Brussels sprouts, remove the outer, tough leaves, and halve the sprouts.

4. Place a steamer insert into a medium saucepan and add water to just below the steamer. Cover and bring the water to a boil over high heat. Add the Brussels sprouts, cover, reduce the heat to medium-high heat, and steam the sprouts for 6 minutes. Transfer the Brussels sprouts to a serving bowl. Pour the sauce over the hot Brussels sprouts, toss, and serve warm or at room temperature, along with toothpicks.

To store: Toss leftover Brussels sprouts in any remaining salsa verde and keep them covered in the refrigerator for 2 days. Serve at room temperature.

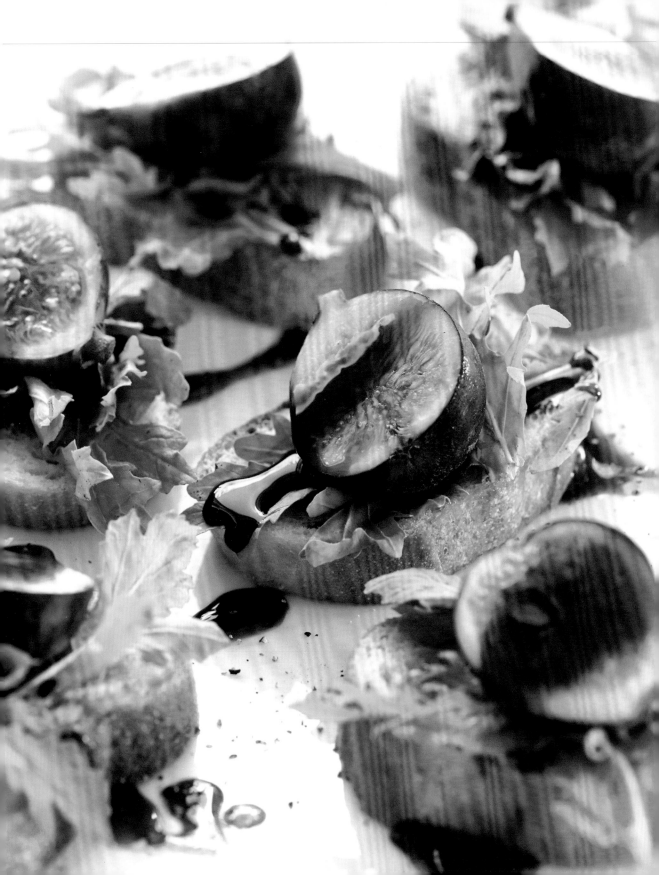

FIG and ARUGULA CROSTINI

MAKES 8 |

Fresh figs caramelized in a bit of butter are exquisite arranged on arugula and drizzled with a honeyed balsamic glaze that makes them glow like jewels. Serve on toasted Italian semolina bread or on salad plates. Finish with some curls of Parmigiano-Reggiano if desired. Black mission figs are best, but use any kind that are plump and juicy. Many supermarkets carry Italian semolina bread.

3 tablespoons balsamic vinegar

1 tablespoon red wine

1 tablespoon honey

8 ½-inch-thick slices Italian semolina bread

1 tablespoon extra-virgin olive oil, plus more for the bread

· · · · · ·

½ packed cup wild arugula, or about the same amount baby arugula

4 ripe black mission figs, halved lengthwise

1 teaspoon unsalted butter

1. Preheat the oven to 350°F.

2. In a small saucepan, boil the vinegar, wine, and honey until you can draw a line with your finger across the back of a spoon coated with the syrupy mixture, about 8 minutes. Set the glaze aside to cool slightly.

3. Meanwhile, arrange the bread slices on a baking sheet. Brush them lightly on one side with oil, then bake until the bread feels firm but is not colored, 8 minutes. Arrange the crostini on a serving platter. Make a bed of arugula on each of the crostini.

4. Trim a thin slice off the rounded side of the halved figs so they can stand firmly. In a skillet, heat the oil and butter over medium-high heat until the butter melts. Add the figs, cut-side down, and cook until they are lightly colored and starting to caramelize, 2 minutes. Place 1 fig half on top of each of the crostini. Brush the figs liberally with the glaze, allowing some to drip onto the arugula. Serve within 30 minutes.

WHITE BEAN and BROCCOLI RABE BRUSCHETTA

SERVES 8 |

Broccoli rabe adds a nice kick to creamy cannellini beans in this easy, light bite. When possible, using a Meyer lemon is nice for its sweeter taste, which comes closest to the flavor that makes the lemons of Campagna and Sicily famous. Serve this bruschetta as part of an antipasto spread for the cocktail hour or make it part of a casual meal, adding a selection of cheeses and a green salad. Grill the bread up to 8 hours ahead and keep it wrapped in foil on the counter, if you like. Vegans can use water in place of chicken broth.

1 bunch broccoli rabe (about 1¼ pounds), woody stems cut off, coarsely chopped

8 ½-inch-thick slices whole-wheat Italian bread

3½ tablespoons extra-virgin olive oil

1 small onion, finely chopped (½ cup)

1 large garlic clove, finely chopped

1 15-ounce can cannellini beans, drained

½ cup fat-free reduced-sodium chicken broth, or water

⅛ teaspoon dried red pepper flakes

½ teaspoon salt

Freshly ground pepper

½ Meyer lemon or regular lemon

1. In a large covered saucepan, boil 6 cups of water. Add the broccoli rabe, pushing it into the water with a wooden spoon. Cook the rabe for 4 minutes over medium-high heat. Drain in a colander, then run cold water over the broccoli rabe while swishing with your hand until the greens feel cool, 30 seconds. Gently squeeze the greens to remove excess water. Finely chop the broccoli rabe, then pull it apart; there will be about 1½ cups.

2. Heat a grill to medium-high or set a ridged grill pan over high heat.

3. Brush the bread slices on one side, using 1 tablespoon of the olive oil. Placing the bread oil side down, grill it until the slices are well marked, about 2 minutes. Turn and grill the bread until marked on the second side, 1 to 2 minutes. Set the grilled bread aside.

4. Heat 1 tablespoon of the remaining oil in a medium skillet over medium-high heat. Add the onion and cook, stirring often, until it is translucent, 4 minutes. Add the garlic and cook until the onion is soft, stirring often, 3 minutes. To avoid the onion and garlic browning, reduce the heat if necessary.

5. Add the beans, chopped broccoli rabe, broth, pepper flakes, and salt to the skillet and cook, stirring occasionally, until the pan is almost dry, 4 minutes. Taking the mixture off

the heat, use a sturdy fork to coarsely mash the beans and greens. Season with pepper and adjust the salt.

6. To serve, top the oil-brushed side of the bread with one-quarter cup of the beans and greens. Drizzle each slice with some of the remaining 1½ tablespoons of oil. Add a few drops of lemon juice, and serve the bruschetta warm.

COOK'S TIP

Rinsing canned beans removes sodium and most of their flavor. Instead, look for reduced-sodium or no-sodium-added beans and simply drain them in a colander.

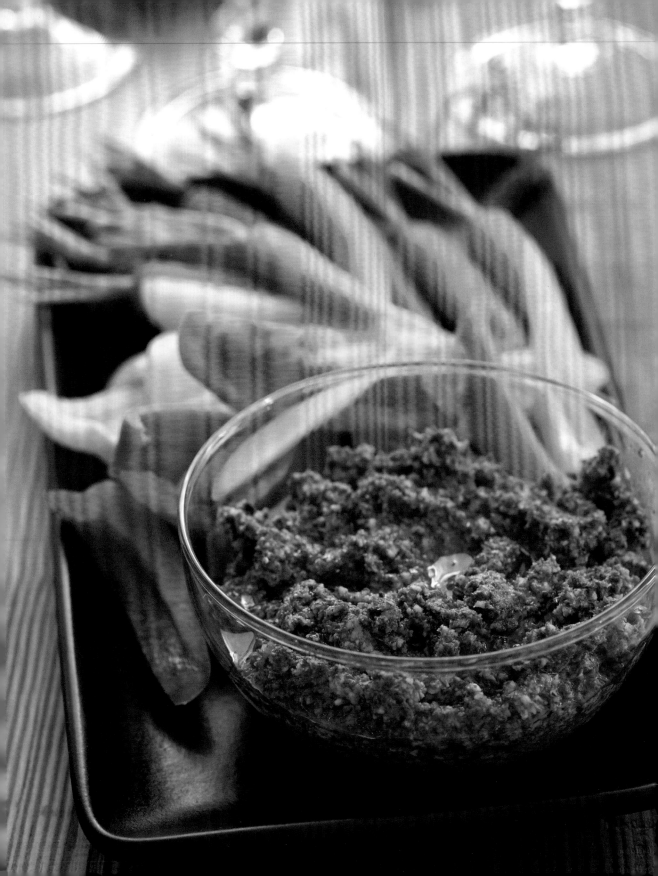

KALE PESTO with CARROT and SWEET PEPPER CRUDITÉS

SERVES 4 |

Raw kale combined with walnuts and pecorino cheese makes a rustic pesto served here as a dip accompanied by sweet pepper strips and carrot sticks for scooping it up. Serve toasted slices of baguette or your favorite crackers with it in addition to the vegetables if you like. This bold pesto is also good mashed with white beans, then spooned onto toasted whole-grain bread for an ad hoc bruschetta. I also mix a dollop of it into lentil soup, toss it with whole-wheat fusilli (first loosening it up with a bit of the pasta cooking water), or for brunch, fill an omelet with thinly sliced Fontina cheese and a generous spoonful of Kale Pesto.

4 large green curly kale leaves, stemmed and chopped (4 packed cups)

2 large garlic cloves, coarsely chopped

¼ cup chopped walnuts

3 tablespoons grated pecorino cheese

⅓ cup extra-virgin olive oil

Salt and freshly ground pepper

3 sweet bell peppers, red, orange, and yellow, seeded and cut into 1-inch strips

1 large carrot, cut into 3-inch by ¼-inch strips

1. In a food processor, pulse the kale, garlic, walnuts, and cheese until the mixture is well combined and looks moist, about 20 pulses. With the motor running, slowly drizzle in the oil in a thin stream. Season with salt and pepper. Let the kale pesto sit for 30 minutes to allow the flavors to meld. Just before serving, taste and adjust the seasoning.

2. To serve, set a bowl with the pesto in the center of a platter or serving board. Arrange the vegetable strips around the bowl of pesto.

To store: Kale Pesto keeps for 5 days with plastic wrap pressed over the top in the refrigerator.

WATERCRESS DEVILED EGGS

MAKES 8 PIECES |

Of all the deviled eggs I have made, this watercress-flecked version disappears fastest. The secret of their appeal is the extra bite added by the cress. For tender-firm whites and perfect, creamy yolks, take time to read how to hard-cook the eggs properly. (See Note below.)

4 hard-cooked eggs, peeled and halved lengthwise, see Note

1 tablespoon light mayonnaise

1 tablespoon light sour cream

1 teaspoon Dijon-style mustard

½ lightly packed cup watercress leaves, finely chopped

2 teaspoons snipped chives

Salt and freshly ground pepper

1. Separate the egg yolks from the whites, arranging the whites on a serving plate and placing the yolks in a small mixing bowl. Add the mayonnaise, sour cream, and mustard to the yolks and mash with a fork until the yolks are creamy. Mix in the watercress and half of the chives. Season the yolks to taste with salt and pepper, being generous with the pepper.

2. Using a small teaspoon, scoop up some of the filling, taking three or four small spoonfuls to fill the cavity, and mound the yolk. With the back of the tip of the spoon, gently smooth the yolk, using a twisting motion to make little peaks and valleys. Repeat to stuff the remaining eggs. Sprinkle a few of the remaining chives on top of each yolk for garnish. Tent foil over the plate of stuffed eggs, and refrigerate them for 1 to 12 hours.

OVEN HARD-COOKED EGGS

Alton Brown uses this method to make the creamiest, best hard-cooked eggs; making just two or a dozen eggs is equally easy.

Preheat the oven to 325°F. Soak a dishtowel and barely wring it out. Spread the towel to cover the oven rack. Arrange room-temperature raw eggs on the rack.

Bake for 30 minutes. Transfer the eggs to a large bowl. Shake them in the bowl to crack them. Fill the bowl with cold water. When the eggs are cool, peel them. They keep in cold water for 3 days. Eggs at least 1 week old peel more easily.

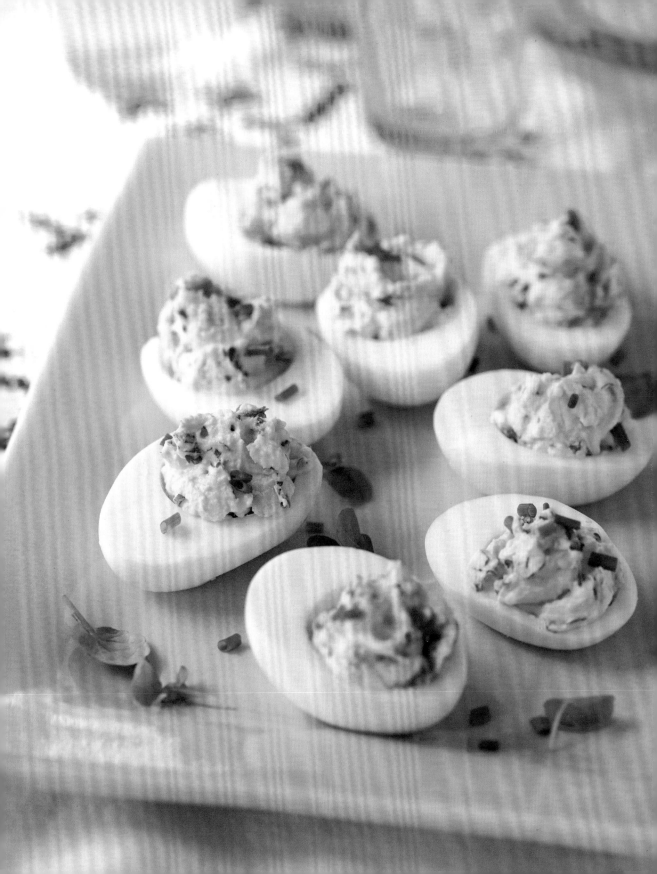

HUMMUS with ARUGULA and PARSLEY

MAKES 1½ CUPS |

Arugula and parsley tint this lemony hummus a fresh green. Keeping it thick lets you scoop it up with pita chips or cucumber slices or stuff it into celery. I also like serving this hummus the Israeli way called *masabacha*, topped with warmed whole chickpeas, a swirl of fruity olive oil, and a dusting of cumin and paprika. Accompanied by warm pita bread it is a light meal. Refrigerate this hummus for 1 to 24 hours before serving, covered with plastic wrap, and it will taste even better.

1 15-ounce can chickpeas, drained, or 1¾ cups cooked chickpeas

½ lightly packed cup wild or baby arugula

½ firmly packed cup flat-leaf parsley leaves

1 scallion, green part only, chopped

1 garlic clove, finely chopped

½ teaspoon ground cumin

3 tablespoons tahini

3 tablespoons fresh lemon juice

2 tablespoons extra-virgin olive oil

Salt and freshly ground pepper

1. In a food processor, pulse the chickpeas to coarsely chop them, 5 pulses. Add the arugula, parsley, scallion, garlic, cumin, tahini, and lemon juice, and pulse until the vegetables are finely chopped, stopping once or twice to scrape down the sides of the bowl.

2. With the motor running, drizzle in the oil, and continue pulsing until it is blended in. If the hummus is too thick, add warm water, 1 tablespoon at a time, until it is spreadable but still slightly grainy. Season the hummus with salt and pepper to taste. Serve the hummus in a bowl, accompanied by chips and cut-up raw vegetables.

To store: This hummus will keep for 3 days tightly covered in the refrigerator.

NUTRINOTE

Canned organic beans do not contain the sulfites used to preserve color in conventional brands. Also, look for cans marked BPA-free to avoid those with a lining that may contain that carcinogen.

MEXICAN SEVEN LAYER DIP

SERVES 12 TO 16 |

This game-day favorite uses lots of avocado, which is full of beneficial fat. To compensate for using generous amounts of sour cream and Jack cheese, the sour cream is reduced-fat and the refried beans are made using minimal oil. Spinach combined with cilantro adds a layer of fresh greens. I serve this dip right away, while the beans are warm, the sour cream cool, and the greens are bright, but if you prefer a divine mess, let the dip sit at room temperature for up to an hour after assembling it. Serve with big, baked tortilla chips.

2 teaspoons canola oil

1 15-ounce can pinto beans, drained

1 teaspoon dried oregano

½ teaspoon ground cumin

½ teaspoon salt

Freshly ground pepper

1 firmly packed cup baby spinach, finely chopped

½ lightly packed cup cilantro leaves, chopped

1 cup bottled salsa, mild or medium hot

1 large Hass avocado, pitted, peeled, and cut into ½-inch cubes

1 cup reduced-fat sour cream

1 cup shredded reduced-fat Monterey Jack cheese (4 ounces)

3 plum tomatoes, halved, seeded, and chopped

2 to 4 tablespoons finely chopped drained canned jalapeño peppers

¼ cup chopped scallions, green part only

1. Lightly coat an 8 x 8 x 2-inch clear glass baking dish or a 2-quart serving bowl with cooking spray and set aside.

2. Heat the oil in a medium skillet over medium-high heat. Add the beans, oregano, cumin, salt, and four grinds of pepper, and stir until the beans are hot. Remove from the heat and use a sturdy fork to mash the beans into a chunky mess, 3 minutes. Spread the beans in the prepared dish in an even layer. Immediately cover them with the chopped spinach and cilantro so the beans do not dry out.

3. Spoon the salsa over the layer of greens. Distribute the avocado over the salsa. Dollop on the sour cream, and with the back of the spoon, gently spread it to cover the avocado. Sprinkle on the shredded cheese. To top off the dip, sprinkle the tomatoes, jalapeños, and scallions over the sour cream. Serve immediately, accompanied by sturdy, large tortilla chips.

GOOD TECHNIQUE

To keep avocado from discoloring, toss it with a teaspoon of fresh lime juice and it will keep in the refrigerator for a day.

NUTRINOTE

Avocado contains monounsaturated fat that can help lower blood cholesterol.

CAPONATA of DARK GREENS

SERVES 4 |

This caponata featuring beet greens and chard that tint it garnet red is as authentic as the traditional one made with eggplant. It still uses the Sicilian *agro-dolce* combination of tomato sauce, olives, sugar, and vinegar. For a full antipasto spread, serve this along with Roasted Red Peppers Stuffed with Kale (p. 31), White Bean and Broccoli Rabe Bruschetta (p. 18), olive-oil-packed tuna, and a generous hunk of pecorino cheese. It is also good as a side dish served with grilled fish and steamed potatoes drizzled with olive oil.

Greens from 1 bunch of beets

4 leaves yellow or rainbow chard

1 tablespoon extra-virgin olive oil

1 medium red onion, halved and cut vertically into thin, crescent-shaped slices

1 celery rib, thinly sliced

½ cup tomato puree

4 pitted Sicilian-style olives, chopped

1 tablespoon white wine vinegar

1 teaspoon sugar

Salt and freshly ground pepper

2 tablespoons slivered almonds or peanuts

1. If the beet stems are thin, cut them off at the base of the leaf. If they are more than ¼-inch thick, Fold and Tear them, holding a leaf in one hand with the stem pointing up and folding the front sides toward each other like closing a book. Working from the base down toward the tip of the leaf, gently tug the leaf away from the center vein. For the chard, tear out the center vein and stem, or cut them out using a V-Cut, laying a leaf on your work surface and running a sharp knife down either side, then lifting away the vein and stem. In a large bowl, rinse the combined greens in several changes of cold water, then drain. Don't worry about water clinging to the leaves.

2. In a large covered saucepan, boil 8 cups of water. Add the greens, pushing them into the water with a wooden spoon. Cook the greens for 2 minutes over medium-high heat. Drain in a colander, then run cold water over the greens while swishing with your hand until the greens feel cool, 30 seconds. Gently squeeze the greens to remove excess water. Finely chop the greens, then pull them apart; there will be about 1½ cups.

3. Heat the oil in a medium skillet over medium-high heat. Add the onion and celery, and cook, stirring often, until the onion is golden, 6 minutes. Add the chopped greens, tomato puree, and ½ cup water. Simmer, stirring occasionally, until most of the moisture is gone and the greens are tender, about 12 minutes. Mix in the olives, vinegar, and sugar, and cook, stirring, for 1 minute. Season with salt and

pepper. Mix in half the nuts. Transfer the caponata to a bowl and set it aside to cool. Before serving, sprinkle on the remaining nuts.

To store: This dish keeps tightly covered in the refrigerator for 4 days.

GOOD TECHNIQUE

Squeezing the greens well ensures that your caponata is not watered down.

SHRIMP with GREEN HERB MAYONNAISE

SERVES 4 |

Chilled shrimp cocktail with spicy red sauce was my favorite combination until French friends introduced me to dipping them in shallot-spiked mayonnaise. Homemade mayonnaise is divine but customizing a top-drawer mayo like Hellmann's or a boutique brand by adding fresh green flavor is nearly as good. Also serve Green Herb Mayonnaise with salmon, use it on Bacon, Arugula, and Tomato on Focaccia (p. 185), and to make egg salad or dress potato salad.

½ cup premium quality mayonnaise, regular or light

¼ teaspoon dry mustard powder

1 teaspoon fresh lemon juice

2 tablespoons finely chopped flat-leaf parsley

1 tablespoon finely chopped baby spinach

2 teaspoons minced chives

1 teaspoon very finely chopped shallots

Freshly ground pepper

1 pound medium-large (36- to 42-count) cooked shrimp, shelled and chilled

1. In a small bowl, whisk together the mayonnaise, mustard powder, and lemon juice. Stir in the parsley, spinach, chives, and shallots. Set aside, or refrigerate for up to 3 days tightly covered in the refrigerator.

2. Arrange the chilled shrimp on a platter, then spoon the mayonnaise into a bowl and add it to the platter. Or divide the shrimp among 4 individual plates, spoon the mayonnaise into four small bowls, and set one on each plate. Serve immediately.

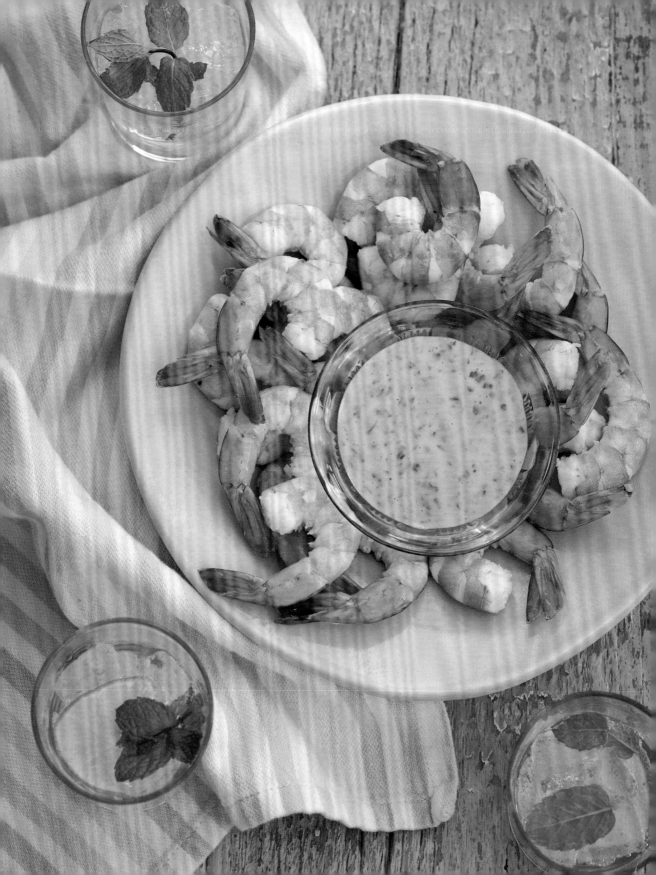

CAYENNE SHORTBREAD with CRISPED KALE

MAKES 36 PIECES |

Rich with cheese and delivering a hint of heat, these golden coins are like super-flaky cheese straws in the round. They come out as tender as puff pastry, but this soft dough is easier to shape and bake. Just remember that chilling it is essential. Crushed Crisped Kale adds a nutty taste to this shortbread's intense cheese flavor. This shortbread goes well with a cold beer, dry white wine, or chilled hard cider.

3/4 cup Crisped Kale (p. 178), preferably Tuscan

8 tablespoons (1 stick) unsalted butter, cut into 16 pieces and chilled

2 cups (8 ounces) shredded Comté or Gruyère cheese

1½ cups unbleached all-purpose flour

1 large egg, lightly beaten

⅛ to ¼ teaspoon cayenne pepper

½ teaspoon salt

NUTRINOTE

Cayenne pepper contains capsaicin, a compound that may help to reduce blood cholesterol as well as fight inflammation.

---

1. A handful at a time, hold the Crisped Kale over a bowl and crush it finely. Using your fingers, work the kale until much of it is about the size of coarsely ground pepper. Some will be as fine as powder. Set the crushed kale aside.

2. In a food processor, pulse the butter, cheese, flour, egg, cayenne, and salt until they combine to resemble coarse meal, about 20 pulses. Turn out the crumbly dough onto a work surface. Sprinkle on the crushed kale, then gather and press the dough gently, distributing the kale evenly as you work the dough just enough to bring it together. It may remain slightly dry.

3. Divide the dough in half, and place each half on a large sheet of wax paper. Use the paper to shape each half into a log about 9 inches long by 1½ inches wide. Repeat with the second half. Wrap the dough in the wax paper and refrigerate for 1 to 24 hours.

4. When ready to bake, preheat the oven to 400°F.

5. Cut the chilled dough into ½-inch slices. Place the slices on a light-colored baking sheet, spacing them 1 inch apart.

6. Bake the shortbread for 20 minutes, or until it is puffed and golden brown. Transfer the shortbread to a wire rack and cool.

To store: This shortbread keeps for 5 days stored in an air-tight tin at room temperature.

ROASTED RED PEPPERS STUFFED with KALE

MAKES 12 ROLLS |

These peppers create a Greek flavor party in your mouth. The idea of pairing sweet peppers with kale comes from Dennis Cotter, the chef at London's Café Paradiso, who elevates vegetarian cooking with his stunning inspirations. Including cheese and nuts in the filling makes these a substantial cocktail accompaniment.

6 large red bell peppers, halved lengthwise, and seeds and ribs removed

½ bunch (about 6 ounces) green kale, cut, rinsed, and stems removed

⅓ cup finely chopped walnuts

¼ cup golden raisins

⅓ cup (1½ ounces) crumbled feta cheese

Salt and freshly ground pepper

1. Set the oven rack to about 4 inches from the heat source. Preheat the broiler. Coat an 8 x 8-inch baking dish with cooking spray.

2. Bring the peppers to room temperature if they are refrigerated. Line a baking sheet with foil. Arrange the peppers, cut side down, on the baking sheet. Place the peppers under the broiler until the skin is blistered and blackened in places, about 6 minutes. Watch the peppers carefully, using tongs to move them on the baking sheet, if necessary. Transfer the peppers to a large bowl, cover with plastic wrap, and let them steam for 20 minutes. With your fingers, remove their skin.

3. While the peppers steam, in a large covered saucepan, boil 4 cups of water. Add the kale, pushing it into the water with a wooden spoon. Cook the kale for 6 minutes over medium-high heat, until it is tender. Drain in a colander, then run cold water over the kale while swishing with your hand until the greens feel cool, 30 seconds. Gently squeeze the greens to remove excess water. Finely chop the kale, then pull it apart; there will be about 1 cup.

4. For the filling, combine the kale, nuts, raisins, and feta in a bowl. Season with salt and pepper.

5. Place a roasted pepper half on a work surface with the bottom toward you. Spoon a generous tablespoon down the center of the pepper. Fold the sides in over the filling; they will overlap slightly at the top and bottom to form a

little boat. Place the filled pepper in the baking dish. Repeat, packing the peppers closely together; there will be space left in the baking dish. Cover the baking dish with foil, sealing it tightly.

6. Bake the filled peppers for 30 minutes. Uncover and cool the peppers in the dish on a wire rack. Serve at room temperature, using a wide spatula to transfer them to a serving dish or individual plates. Or cover with plastic wrap and refrigerate the peppers for up to 24 hours. Let stand until room temperature before serving.

To store: This dish keeps covered in the refrigerator for 4 days.

NUTRINOTE

Red bell peppers are loaded with vitamin A, which helps keep your lungs and digestive tract healthy.

COLLARD GREEN DOLMAS FILLED with WILD RICE and SUN-DRIED TOMATO PESTO

MAKES 16 PIECES: 8 SERVINGS AS AN ANTIPASTO, 4 SERVINGS AS A LIGHT MEAL |

At parties, these stuffed collard rolls disappear even faster than a platter of shrimp. The flavor of tomato pesto sweetens the collard's taste and complements the earthiness of the rice. Trimming the leaves almost into rectangles makes filling and rolling them quick and efficient. Serve these rolls individually as a finger food or pair them with Roasted Red Peppers Stuffed with Kale (p. 31) and Italian *salume* for a casual meal. To make them vegan, I use Seggiano's sun-dried tomato pesto and add a touch of sweet mellow miso to replace the kick of aged cheese.

⅓ cup wild rice

8 large collard leaves

3 tablespoons prepared sun-dried tomato pesto

Salt and freshly ground pepper

1 tablespoon extra-virgin olive oil

½ cup fat-free reduced-sodium chicken broth or vegetable broth

1. Preheat the oven to 350°F. Coat an 8-inch square baking dish with cooking spray or brush it with olive oil, and set aside.

2. In a covered medium saucepan, cook the wild rice with 1¾ cups water until it is very tender, 50 to 60 minutes. Set the covered rice aside for 10 minutes. Using a fork, fluff the rice. Transfer the rice to a mixing bowl to cool.

3. Meanwhile, fill a large pot with water, cover, and bring it to a boil over high heat.

4. While the water boils, prepare the collard leaves: Make a V-Cut and lift out the center vein and stem from the leaves. Slit the leaves to the tip, making 16 halves. Stacking 3 or 4 halves with the long, straight side toward you, trim the collards at both ends to make 8-inch rectangles curved at the top edge. They will vary in height, which does not matter.

5. Cook the collard leaves in the boiling water until almost tender, 8 to 10 minutes, reducing the heat to medium-high. Using tongs, transfer the leaves to a large bowl and cool

continued on page 35

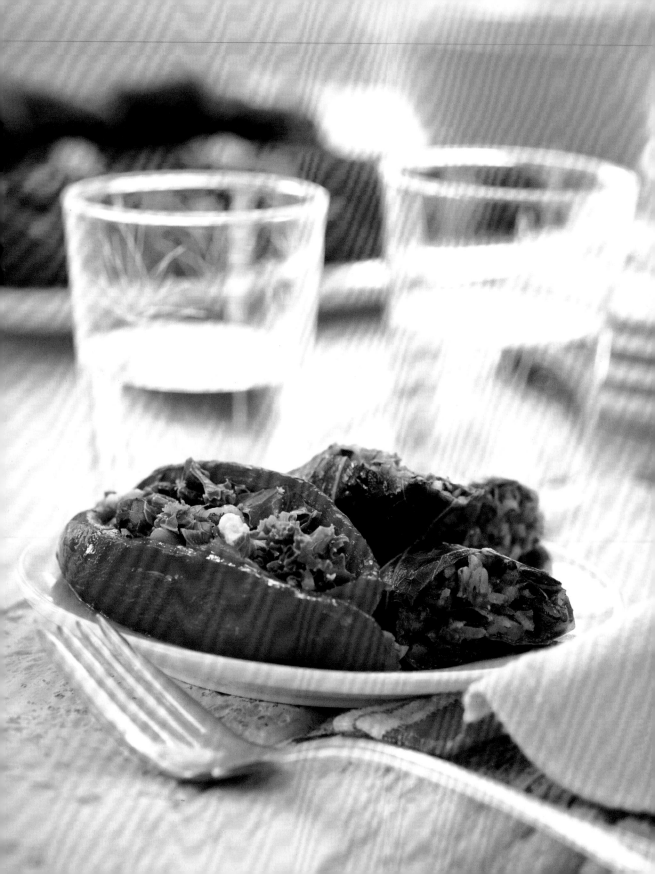

them under running cold water. Pat the leaves thoroughly dry with paper towels.

6. For the filling, combine the pesto and wild rice, and season with salt and pepper to taste.

7. Lay a collard leaf on a work surface with the curved top facing away from you. Place a generous tablespoon of the filling an inch above the bottom of the leaf, in the center, smoothing it with the back of the spoon into a 2-inch square. Fold in one side of the leaf to cover the filling. Fold in the other side. Lift up the bottom edge, and roll away from you while pushing the filling toward you to help pack it; the filled collard will resemble a stuffed grape leaf. Place the stuffed collard in the prepared baking dish. Repeat, packing the baking dish tightly with the stuffed leaves. I usually make two rows plus a few fitted in along one side.

At this point, the unbaked stuffed leaves can be refrigerated overnight in a covered baking dish. Bring them to room temperature and brush with oil before baking.

8. Brush the olive oil over the stuffed rolls. Pour in the broth. Cover the baking dish with foil, sealing it tightly. Bake the stuffed collards for 30 minutes. Carefully remove the foil; steam will be released. Cool the collard rolls to room temperature in the pan. To serve, use a wide spatula to transfer the stuffed collard leaves to a serving platter or individual plates.

To store: The baked rolls keep for 3 days covered in the refrigerator. Bring them to room temperature before serving.

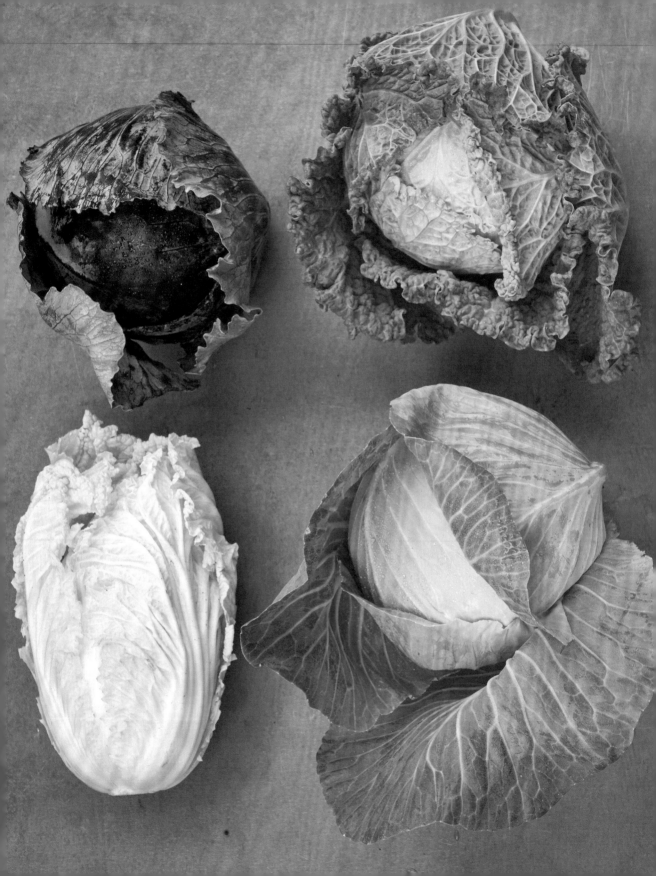

3.

SOUPS

MY GRANDMOTHER MADE THE BEST SOUP IN THE WORLD. Maybe yours did, too, but it was not my grandmother's borscht. She filled the kettle with so many vegetables that they barely had room to swim. With that as my ideal, many of the soups in this chapter are more solid than liquid.

My grandmother, unusually ahead of her time, was mostly vegetarian, but all her soups were so intense and satisfying that I never missed the meat. Happily, my mother made great chicken soup, so that is also part of my soup consciousness.

From thick pea soup for dinner to icy, sharp, watercress soup that my mother made when it was so hot no one wanted to eat, we had soup nearly every day. Belonging to a tribe of health nuts with eclectic tastes, I became comfortable using all kinds of greens. I got ideas for soups using Napa cabbage and bok choy, and kale, too, which was a nearly unknown green back then. I had a wonderful time drawing on all this in creating the fourteen soups here, using twelve kinds of greens and including a veritable bazaar of spices and herbs, including turmeric, caraway seeds, dill, sage, and rosemary.

You can make a meal out of most of these soups, and many of them are meatless, or will be vegan if you simply replace their chicken broth with vegetable broth or water. You will still get plenty of protein from beans, lentils, and the greens, too, since kale, collards, mustard greens, and spinach all provide at least three grams of protein per serving.

Making stock ranks low on my to-do list but most commercially made vegetable broths make soups look carrot orange, bitter-tasting, and full of sodium. So I created The Best Vegetable Stock (p. 58). Make it and see how much better your soups will be.

I use chicken broth in soups where its flavor feels right to me. Vegetable broth alters their flavor, making them differently enjoyable for vegetarians and vegans.

CABBAGE and BRUSSELS SPROUTS SOUP

SERVES 6 |

This wintery soup gets its old-world flavor from caraway seeds, which remind me of the cabbage soup my grandmother made. But in place of her long, slow cooking, I maximize flavor by sweating the vegetables, making this soup ready to serve in under an hour. A thick slab of buttered pumpernickel or sturdy Russian-style rye bread is the perfect accompaniment. Combining commercially made broth with water reduces sodium content as it also allows other flavors to stand out better. Vegans can use vegetable broth.

⅓ small Savoy or green cabbage, about ½ pound

2 tablespoons extra-virgin olive oil

1 pound Brussels sprouts, stem end trimmed, cut crosswise into 4 rounds

1 large onion, peeled and cubed

1 medium carrot, chopped

1 celery rib, sliced crosswise

1 medium white turnip, peeled and cubed, optional

1 small parsnip, peeled and chopped

1 medium Granny Smith apple, peeled, cored, and chopped

½ cup chopped flat-leaf parsley

½ teaspoon caraway seeds

1 dried clove

4 cups fat-free reduced-sodium chicken broth, or vegetable broth

1 medium yellow-flesh potato (6 ounces), peeled and cubed

1 large lemon, ends removed, cut into 6 slices, and seeded

Chopped fresh dill, optional, for garnish

1. Cut the cabbage vertically into 2 or 3 wedges. Cut away the core and thinly slice the wedges crosswise, making 3 cups shredded cabbage.

2. In a large Dutch oven, heat the oil over medium-high heat. Add the cabbage, Brussels sprouts, and onion and cook, stirring often, until the cabbage and sprouts are bright green and look moist, 4 to 5 minutes. Mix in the carrot, celery, turnip, parsnip, and apple, and cook, stirring occasionally, until the cabbage is limp, 4 minutes.

3. Cover, reduce the heat to medium, and let the vegetables sweat for 10 minutes, reducing the heat to avoid browning, if necessary. Mix in the parsley, caraway seeds, and clove.

4. Add the broth and 2 cups water. When the liquid boils, reduce the heat, cover, and simmer the soup for 15 minutes. Add the potato and simmer, covered, until all the vegetables are tender, about 15 minutes.

5. To serve, divide the soup among six wide, shallow bowls. Float a lemon slice in each bowl. If desired, sprinkle some chopped dill into each bowl. This soup keeps for 5 days, covered in the refrigerator. Reheat it in a covered saucepan over medium heat, stirring occasionally.

RIBBOLITA with TUSCAN KALE

SERVES 8 |

Italian cooks make a big pot of this bean soup, serve half of it for dinner, then reheat the rest the next day and serve it ladled over toasted bread. This second heating is why Italians call this soup ribbolita, meaning recooked. Simmering a piece of rind from Parmigiano-Reggiano cheese in the soup, a practice of thrifty Italian cooks, enriches the flavor without using broth. To vary the soup's flavor when serving the second half, I spread the bread with Rosemary Walnut Pesto (p. 42).

1 large carrot, chopped

1 large celery rib, chopped

1 large red onion, diced

3 tablespoons extra-virgin olive oil

2 garlic cloves, chopped

1 medium bunch Tuscan kale (12 ounces), stemmed and cut into ¾-inch ribbons

1 cup butternut squash, diced

2 teaspoons rubbed sage

4-inch by 4-inch piece Parmigiano-Reggiano cheese rind, optional

1 15-ounce can borlotti or red kidney beans, drained, or 1½ cups cooked fresh cranberry beans

Salt and freshly ground pepper

8 1-inch-thick slices whole-wheat Italian bread, grilled or toasted

1. In a food processor, pulse the carrot, celery, and onion until finely chopped and moist.

2. In a large Dutch oven, heat the oil over medium-high heat. Sauté the chopped vegetables until the onion is soft, 6 minutes. Mix in the garlic and cook until the mixture is golden, 3 minutes longer.

3. Mix in the kale until it wilts, 3 minutes, doing this in two additions, if necessary. Pour in 7 cups of cold water. Partially cover the pot, bring the soup to a boil, reduce the heat, and simmer for 10 minutes. Add the squash, sage, and cheese rind, if using. Simmer, uncovered, until the squash is tender, 15 minutes. Add the beans and cook until they are heated through, 5 minutes. Season the soup to taste with salt and pepper.

4. Divide half the soup among four wide, shallow soup bowls. Divide the cheese rind with a large spoon and add a piece to each bowl. Serve immediately. Cool the remaining soup, cover, and refrigerate it overnight.

5. When ready to serve the remaining soup, reheat it covered, over medium heat. Meanwhile, spread 1 tablespoon of Rosemary Walnut Pesto over each grilled bread slice and place it in the bottom of a wide, shallow soup bowl. Ladle the hot soup over the bread and serve.

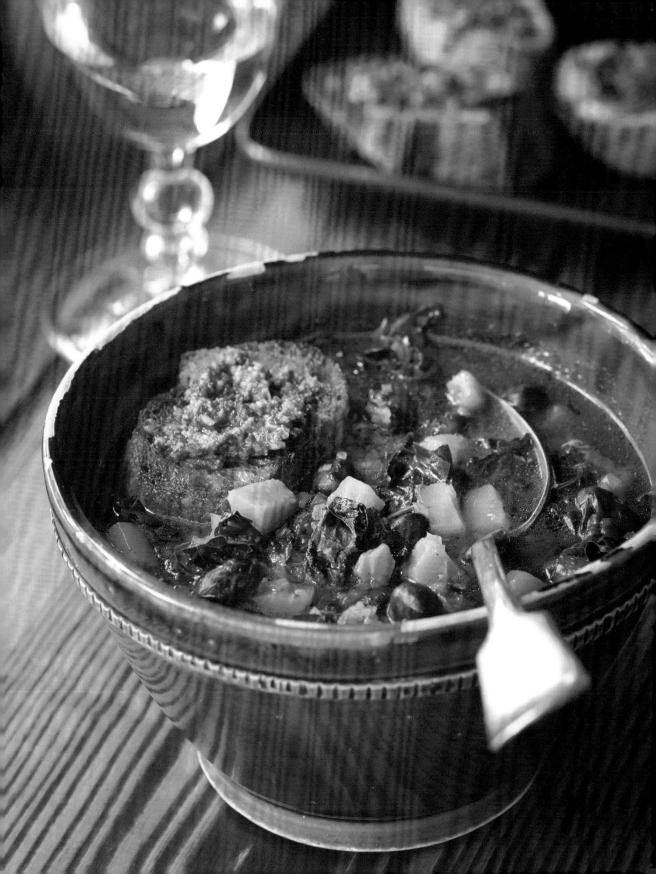

ROSEMARY WALNUT PESTO

In addition to a spread for toasted bread, a spoonful of this pesto enhances green pea soup. I also mix it into warm rice or cooked lentils or combine it with whole-wheat pasta and chickpeas, making a hearty vegetarian dinner.

¼ cup walnuts

8 large basil leaves, torn in pieces

¼ packed cup flat-leaf parsley leaves

1 tablespoon chopped fresh rosemary needles

1 tablespoon fresh thyme leaves

2 tablespoons extra-virgin olive oil

Salt and freshly ground pepper

In a food processor, whirl the walnuts until they are coarsely chopped, 15 seconds. Add the basil, parsley, rosemary, and thyme, and pulse 5 or 6 times. With the motor running, drizzle in the oil; there will be about ¼ cup pesto. Season with salt and pepper.

BLACK LENTIL SOUP with CHARD

SERVES 4 |

Small black lentils, also called beluga or caviar lentils, hold their shape and stay creamy no matter how long they cook. This assures good body in this soup, which includes leafy chard, sweet red pepper, and an aromatic bay leaf. Ladling the hot soup over fresh basil releases its flavor. Feta cheese and balsamic vinegar add Mediterranean accents. Vegans can skip the feta cheese.

1 cup black lentils

1 large bay leaf

1 large leek, white part only, halved lengthwise, and thinly sliced crosswise

1 medium red onion, chopped (1 cup)

1 medium red bell pepper, seeded and chopped

2 large red chard leaves, center ribs and stems removed

4 large fresh basil leaves

¼ cup crumbled feta cheese (2 ounces)

2 teaspoons balsamic vinegar, optional

Salt and freshly ground pepper

1. In a large heavy saucepan, combine the lentils and bay leaf with 5 cups of water. Bring to a boil over medium-high heat, reduce the heat to a simmer, cover, and cook the lentils for 20 minutes.

2. Add the leek, onion, and bell pepper, and simmer the soup, covered, for 10 minutes.

3. While the soup simmers, stack the chard leaves on your work surface and roll the leaves into a long tube. Cut the roll crosswise into ¾-inch strips. Gather the sliced chard into a heap and chop it coarsely; there will be about 3 cups. Add the chard to the soup, cover, and cook until it is tender, about 15 minutes. Season with salt and pepper.

4. To serve, stack the basil leaves, roll them into a tube, and cut them crosswise into thin shreds. Divide the basil among four soup bowls and ladle in the soup. Sprinkle on the feta cheese. Drizzle on the balsamic vinegar, if using. This soup keeps for 4 days tightly covered in the refrigerator. Reheat it in a covered saucepan over medium heat, stirring once or twice.

NUTRINOTE

The acid in balsamic vinegar helps your body utilize the iron in the spinach.

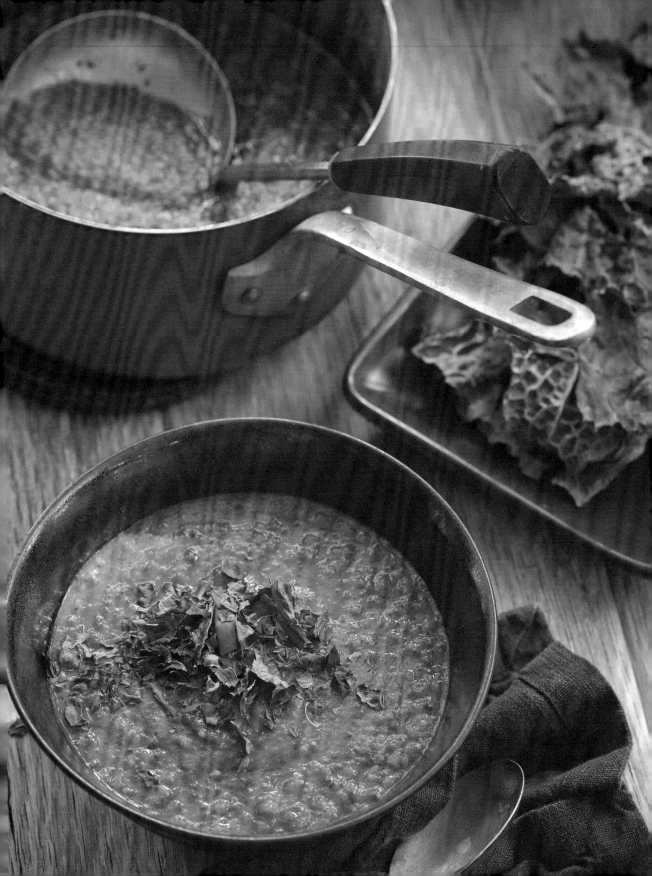

ROASTED TOMATO SOUP with CRISPED COLLARD GREENS

SERVES 4 |

Canned roasted tomatoes give this full-bodied soup a hint of smoke. Warmed by Moroccan spices, this soup comforts your spirit as it nurtures your body. A sprinkling of Crisped Collard Greens (p. 178) is not merely fanciful. Along with crunch, it adds the nutrition of leafy greens.

1 large onion, chopped

3 garlic cloves, unpeeled

2 tablespoons extra-virgin olive oil, divided

2 teaspoons ground cumin

½ teaspoon ground coriander

½ teaspoon ground turmeric

1 large beefsteak-type tomato, seeded and chopped

1 28-ounce can roasted tomatoes

⅛ teaspoon sugar

1 cup vegetable broth

Salt and freshly ground pepper

1 cup Crisped Collard Greens (p. 178)

NUTRINOTE

I add turmeric anywhere its flavor blends in because of its potent antioxidant benefits, always using a judicious amount that harmonizes with a dish's other flavors.

---

1. Preheat the oven to 400°F.

2. On a baking sheet, combine half the onion and all the garlic cloves and coat with 1 tablespoon of the oil. Roast for 25 minutes, stirring after 12 minutes. The garlic will be soft and the onion browned in places. When cool enough to handle, peel the garlic.

3. In a large saucepan, heat the remaining 1 tablespoon oil over medium-high heat. Add the remaining onion and cook, stirring, until it is soft, 5 minutes. Mix in the roasted onion and garlic, then the cumin, coriander, and turmeric, stirring until the spices are fragrant, 30 seconds. Add the chopped tomato, stirring until it breaks down, 5 minutes. Add the canned tomatoes with their liquid, the sugar, and the broth. Cover and simmer until the tomatoes are very tender, 20 minutes. Uncover and let the soup cool for 10 minutes.

4. Transfer the soup to a blender or a super blender, which gives it the creamiest texture, and whirl to puree. Season with salt and pepper.

5. To serve, divide the soup among four wide, shallow soup bowls. Holding one-fourth of the Crisped Collard Greens over the bowl, crush the crisp greens and let them fall on the soup. Serve immediately.

To store: This soup keeps for 5 days tightly covered in the refrigerator. Reheat it in a covered saucepan over medium heat.

ROOT VEGETABLE CHOWDER with KALE

SERVES 4 |

I start making this soup in the fall, when the markets still have sun-warmed local sweet peppers and the first winter squash has arrived. Use chard, collards, or broccoli rabe for the greens, if you wish, and a turnip or a few red radishes in place of the daikon. Add kidney beans, cooked barley, or quinoa to make it a main dish soup. Vegans can use vegetable broth.

1 tablespoon virgin coconut oil

1½ cups butternut squash, peeled and diced

1 large red onion, chopped (1 cup)

3 inches daikon radish, peeled and cut into ¾-inch cubes (¾ cup)

½ large red bell pepper, diced (1 cup)

1 medium carrot, chopped (½ cup)

1 medium parsnip, peeled and chopped (¾ cup)

3 green kale leaves, stems and center veins removed

4 cups fat-free reduced-sodium chicken broth, or vegetable broth

1 medium yellow-fleshed potato, diced

Salt and freshly ground pepper

1. In a large saucepan, heat the oil over medium-high heat. Add the squash, onion, radish, red pepper, carrot, and parsnip, stirring to coat them with the oil. Cook for 5 minutes, stirring occasionally. Cover tightly, reduce the heat to medium-low, and cook for 5 minutes, until the vegetables release their juices.

2. Meanwhile, in a covered large saucepan, boil 1 inch of water over high heat. Add the kale, using a wooden spoon to push it into the water. Reduce the heat to medium-high, cover, and cook for 4 minutes. Drain the kale in a colander and then run cold water over it until cooled, 1 minute, swishing the leaves with your hand. Gently squeeze to remove excess moisture from the kale. Chop the kale into bite-size pieces.

3. Add the broth, potato, and kale to the vegetables. When the broth starts to bubble, cover, reduce the heat, and simmer the soup for 10 minutes, until the vegetables are very tender but not falling apart. Season with salt and pepper. To serve, divide the soup among four wide, shallow bowls.

To store: This soup keeps covered in the refrigerator for 4 days. Reheat leftovers in a covered pot over medium heat.

NUTRINOTE

Yukon Gold potatoes get their color from antioxidant carotenoids.

HOPPIN' JOHN STEW with MUSTARD GREENS

SERVES 4 |

Southerners serve this rice and bean dish on New Year's Day to attract prosperity. I happily make this meatless version throughout the year. This substantial stew may or may not make you wealthy, but its black-eyed peas, red quinoa, and mustard greens will surely make you healthier. Wiser, too, by starting a positive friendship with this super green rarely appreciated outside the South. Collard greens Short Cooked for 5 minutes can replace the mustard greens if you wish (see p. 7).

1 small bunch mustard greens (8 to 9 ounces), stemmed

4 teaspoons canola oil

¾ cup chopped red onion

1 large garlic clove, chopped

1 celery rib, chopped

1 small green bell pepper, seeded and chopped

1 medium jalapeño pepper, seeded and finely chopped

1 15½-ounce can black-eyed peas, drained

1 teaspoon dried thyme

4 cups vegetable broth

1 cup cooked red quinoa

¼ teaspoon smoked paprika

2 teaspoons cider vinegar

Salt and freshly ground pepper

NUTRINOTE

Smoked paprika adds lycopene and great taste as it keeps this Southern stew vegan.

---

1. In a large covered saucepan, boil 4 cups of water. Add the greens, pushing them into the water with a wooden spoon. Cook the greens for 3 minutes over medium-high heat. Drain in a colander, then run cold water over them while swishing with your hand until the greens feel cool, 30 seconds. Gently squeeze the greens to remove excess water. Finely chop the greens, then pull them apart; there will be about 2 cups.

2. In a small Dutch oven or heavy large saucepan, heat the oil over medium-high heat. Add the onion and cook, stirring often, until it is translucent, 4 minutes. Mix in the garlic, celery, green pepper, and jalapeño and cook, stirring often, until the celery begins to soften, 4 minutes.

3. Add the black-eyed peas, thyme, chopped mustard greens, broth, and 2 cups water. Bring the liquid to a boil, reduce the heat, and simmer until the greens are almost tender, 10 minutes.

4. Mix in the quinoa, paprika, and vinegar and cook until the quinoa is heated through, 10 minutes. Season with salt and pepper. To serve, ladle the hot stew into four deep bowls.

To store: This stew keeps for 4 days tightly covered in the refrigerator. Reheat it in a covered saucepan over medium heat, stirring three or four times.

AVGOLEMONO SOUP
with ARUGULA

SERVES 4

Arugula in this lemony chicken and rice soup is so good that I wish I had thought of adding it sooner. To save time, you can start with step 3, using store-bought broth and chicken. The result tastes milder but delivers all the comfort that makes this creamy soup a Greek classic.

1 6-ounce skinless and boneless chicken breast

4 cups fat-free reduced-sodium chicken broth

½ cup long-grain white rice

½ cup chopped arugula

⅓ cup chopped fresh dill

1 large egg, at room temperature

¼ cup fresh lemon juice

Salt and freshly ground pepper

1 teaspoon grated lemon zest, optional, for garnish

1. In a large saucepan, gently simmer the chicken breast in the broth until the chicken is white in the center at its thickest point when tested with a knife, 15 to 20 minutes. When the chicken is cool enough to handle, shred it into bite-size pieces. Reserve 1 cup, and save the rest of the chicken for another use.

2. Line a strainer with cheesecloth or a large coffee filter and set the strainer over a bowl. Strain the broth into the bowl, tilting to help the broth drain; there should be 3¾ cups liquid. Discard the filter and rinse out the saucepan.

3. Return the strained broth to the saucepan or, if using prepared chicken, add the 4 cups of broth, the rice, arugula, and half the dill. Bring the broth to a boil, then simmer, covered, until the rice is soft, 15 minutes.

4. Meanwhile, in a medium bowl, beat the egg, then whisk in the lemon juice and 2 tablespoons water.

5. When the rice is tender, off the heat, pour 1 cup of the hot soup into a measuring cup. Slowly pour this hot soup into the egg-lemon mixture, whisking constantly. Return the egg mixture to the saucepan. Season with salt and pepper.

6. To serve, divide the hot soup among four soup bowls. Add shredded chicken and some of the remaining dill to each bowl. Sprinkle with the lemon zest, if using.

To store: This soup keeps for three days tightly covered in the refrigerator. Reheat it gently, uncovered, over medium heat.

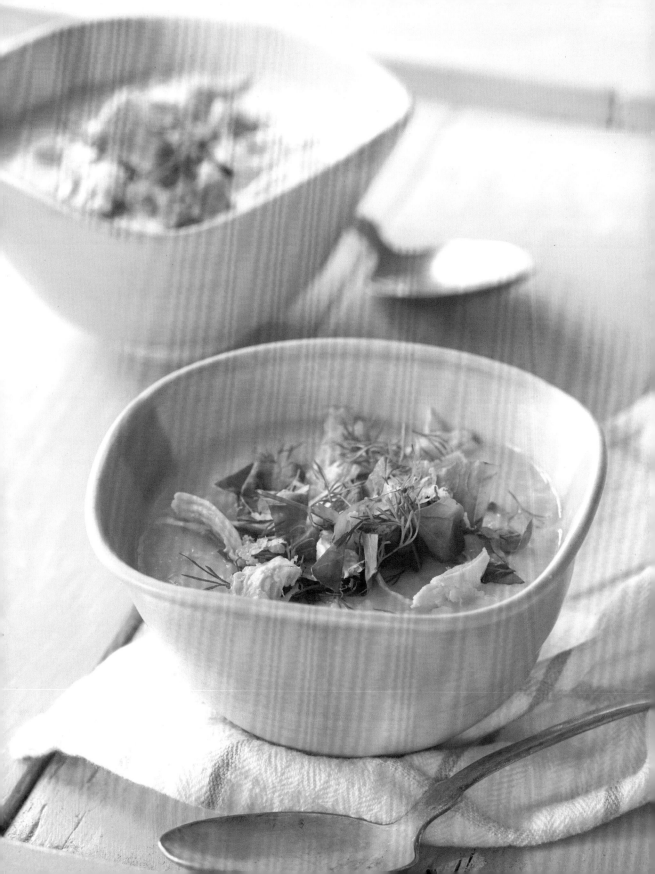

MULLIGATAWNY SOUP with MUSTARD GREENS

SERVES 4 |

When the British ruled India under the Raj, they turned red lentil dal into this soup and added chicken. Here, keeping it vegan, I use coconut oil and milk to bring richness. Garnished with mustard greens, which are widely used in India, chopped apple, and fresh tomato, and accompanied by warm pita bread or fluffy naan, this protein-rich soup makes a complete meal. If you like Indian curries or boldly flavored soups, this is your dish.

1 cup red lentils

1 tablespoon coconut oil

1 cup chopped onion

1 garlic clove, chopped

2 teaspoons curry powder, mild or hot

1 teaspoon ground turmeric

3 cups vegetable broth

6 large mustard green leaves, about 7 ounces, stems and tough central core removed

1 large plum tomato, halved, seeded, and chopped

¼ Granny Smith apple, chopped

¾ cup light coconut milk

Salt and freshly ground pepper

1. Place the lentils in a large bowl. Half fill the bowl with water, use your fingers to swish the lentils, then pour out the cloudy water. The wet lentils clump together so keeping them in the bowl is easy. Repeat, rinsing the lentils three or four times, until the water runs almost clear.

2. In a large saucepan, heat the coconut oil over medium-high heat. Add the onion and cook until it is translucent, 4 minutes, stirring often. Add the garlic and cook 1 minute. Mix in the curry powder and turmeric, stirring to coat the onion. Add the lentils, broth, and 2 cups water. Bring to a boil, reduce the heat, and simmer, covered, until the lentils are soft, 20 minutes.

3. Meanwhile, in a covered, large saucepan, boil 2 inches of cold water over high heat. Add the mustard greens and cook for 3 minutes to collapse and soften the leaves. Immediately, use tongs to transfer the mustard greens to a bowl and set the bowl in the sink under cold running water. Swish the greens with your hands until they are cooled, 30 seconds. Gather up the greens and squeeze out the excess moisture; you may need to do this in two handfuls. Finely chop the mustard greens, then pull them apart; there will be about 1 cup.

4. For the garnish, combine the chopped mustard greens, tomato, and apple in a bowl. Heat ¼ cup of the coconut milk in a medium skillet over medium-high heat until it

bubbles, 1 minute. Add the mustard greens mixture and cook, stirring occasionally, until it is heated through, 3 minutes.

5. Finish the soup by pureeing it with an immersion blender or whirling it in a blender. Blend in the remaining ½ cup coconut milk. Season with salt and pepper. Serve the soup in four wide, shallow bowls, with one-fourth of the warm mustard greens mounded in the center of each.

To store: This soup keeps in the refrigerator for 4 days tightly covered. Reheat it in a covered saucepan over medium heat, stirring two or three times.

GOOD TECHNIQUE

Red lentils do not require soaking but they need a thorough washing to eliminate fine dust clinging to them that can make a dish gritty. Visible only as you rinse the lentils, this dust requires several changes of water to eliminate it.

HOT and SOUR SOUP with BOK CHOY

SERVES 4

The flavors in this soup hit you in waves, starting with pungent cilantro, followed by earthy mushrooms and then toasted sesame. Next, tingling heat and vinegar sharpness make your taste buds buzz. Finally, this flavor commotion winds down so you taste the creamy tofu. While the mushrooms are soaking, measure, chop, and combine the other ingredients, and this umami-loaded soup is ready to serve in 10 minutes.

4 dried Chinese or shiitake mushrooms (see Note)

1/2 cup canned shredded bamboo shoots

2 tablespoons cornstarch

1 teaspoon sugar

1/2 teaspoon salt

2 tablespoons rice wine vinegar

1 tablespoon red wine vinegar

1 1/2 teaspoons reduced-sodium soy sauce

1 large egg

1 teaspoon toasted sesame oil

1 tablespoon peanut oil

2 ribs bok choy, white part only, thinly sliced crosswise

4 cups fat-free reduced-sodium chicken broth

3 1/2 to 4 3/4 ounces firm tofu (1/4 of 14- to 15-ounce package), cut into 3/4-inch cubes

1/2 teaspoon ground white pepper

2 tablespoons coarsely chopped cilantro

2 tablespoons chopped scallions, green part only

1. In a bowl, soak the mushrooms in 1 1/2 cups hot tap water until softened, 20 to 30 minutes. Cut off and discard the stems. Cut the mushrooms into thin strips. Measure and save 1 cup of the soaking liquid.

2. While the mushrooms soak, in a small saucepan cover the bamboo shoots with cold water to a depth of 1 inch. Cook over medium-high heat until the water boils, then drain and set the bamboo shoots aside.

3. In a small bowl, combine the cornstarch, sugar, salt, rice and red wine vinegars, and soy sauce, whisking until the sugar and salt dissolve. In another bowl, beat the egg with the sesame oil.

4. In a large saucepan, heat the peanut oil over medium-high heat. Add the bok choy, bamboo shoots, and mushrooms and cook, stirring, for 1 minute. Add the broth and reserved mushroom liquid. When the liquid boils, add the tofu, and reduce the heat to a simmer. Restir the cornstarch mixture, then add it into the soup, whisking until the soup looks clear, 2 minutes.

5. While whisking briskly in one direction, slowly drizzle in the beaten egg. Add the pepper.

6. To serve, divide the soup among four deep bowls. Garnish each bowl with one-fourth of the cilantro and scallions.

To store: Cover leftovers and refrigerate overnight, then serve at room temperature the next day.

MUSHROOM MATTERS

Dried mushrooms are fundamental to the flavor in hot and sour soup. Use fleshy Chinese black mushrooms, lighter colored golden oak mushrooms, or Japanese dried shiitake mushrooms.

Soak the mushrooms in very hot tap water rather than boiling water to release more of their flavor. They float, so use a wide, shallow bowl and set a plate that fits inside the bowl over them to hold the mushrooms down. Or, flip the mushrooms over three or four times while they soak.

THAI COCONUT SOUP with SHRIMP and SAVOY CABBAGE

SERVES 4 | (GF)

You can make this soup, topped with shrimp and dense with vegetables, blazing hot or delicately mild. I rarely suggest making a special broth but the infusion of daikon radish, fresh basil, and ginger that is the base for this soup is worth doing. Prepare it several days ahead or set it to simmer while you prep the soup's other ingredients, and then finish the soup using the same pot.

ASIAN BROTH

5 inches daikon radish, chopped (1 cup)

1 medium onion, chopped (1 cup)

1 scallion, white part only, sliced

8 cilantro sprigs, stems included

6 stems from fresh Thai or Italian basil

½ inch fresh ginger, sliced

. . . . . .

8 ounces Savoy cabbage (⅓ of a small head)

1 medium onion

3 garlic cloves

½ inch fresh ginger

1 red or green hot chile pepper

2½ inches fresh lemongrass

1 tablespoon coconut oil

1 cup light coconut milk

1 tablespoon good quality fish sauce, such as Thai Kitchen

3 ounces small cremini mushrooms

12 (16- to 20-count) shrimp, cooked and shelled

¼ cup cilantro leaves, for garnish

1. For the broth, in a large saucepan, combine the daikon, onion, scallion, cilantro, basil stems, and ginger with 4 cups of water. Bring just to a boil, uncovered, then reduce the heat and simmer for 15 minutes. Strain the broth into a bowl, discarding the solids; wipe out the pot. There will be 4 cups broth; it keeps tightly covered in the refrigerator for up to 5 days.

2. While the broth simmers, cut the cabbage into 2-inch wedges, then slice the wedges crosswise into ½-inch strips. Cut the onion into thin crescents. Thinly slice the garlic and ginger. Slice the chile pepper, discarding the seeds, if desired. Smash the lemongrass with the side of a heavy knife or a mallet to bruise it.

3. In the saucepan from the broth, heat the coconut oil over medium-high heat. Add the cabbage, onion, garlic, ginger, chile pepper, and lemongrass, and cook until cabbage is limp, 4 minutes, stirring occasionally. Add 3 cups of the broth and simmer until the cabbage is almost tender, 5 minutes. Reserve the remaining broth for another use. Add the coconut milk, fish sauce, and mushrooms, and simmer until the cabbage is tender, 3 minutes.

4. To serve, divide the soup among four bowls. Add the shrimp and garnish with the cilantro.

To store: Store leftovers tightly covered in the refrigerator for 3 days. Reheat the soup gently in an uncovered saucepan over medium heat, stirring occasionally.

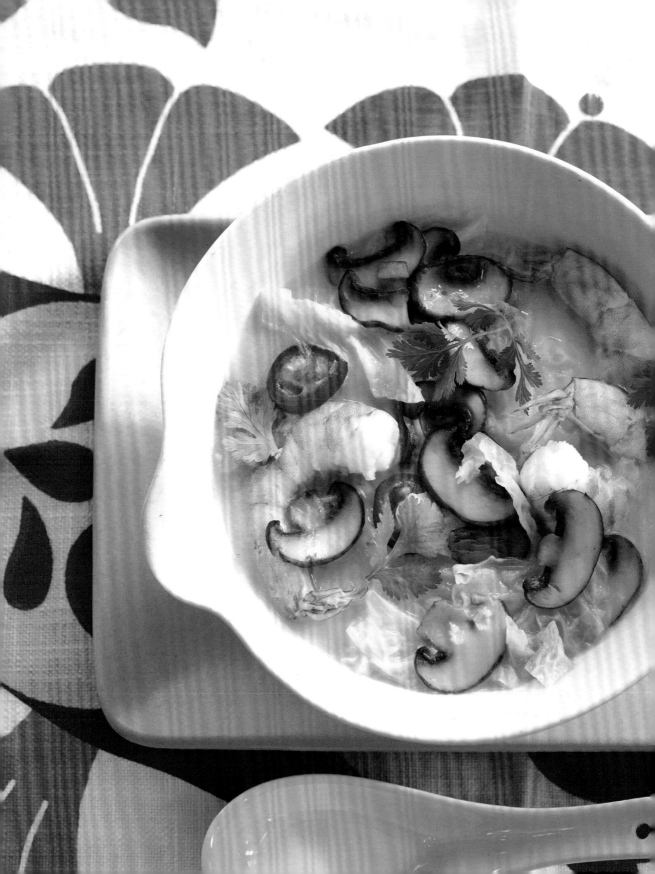

CHILLED WATERCRESS SOUP

SERVES 4 | (GF)

Watercress makes this dark green soup sharply refreshing. Serving it with a float of heavy cream on top uses a little fat—just a spoonful—to maximum effect. Whip the rest of the cream and serve it with fresh berries or a fruit crisp for dessert, if you like.

1 bunch watercress (5 to 6 ounces), or 1 (4-ounce) bag

1 small onion, chopped (½ cup)

1 tablespoon long-grain white rice

1 cup fat-free reduced-sodium chicken broth

Salt and freshly ground pepper

4 tablespoons heavy cream

2 tablespoons snipped chives

1. Separate the leafy tips and thin, tender upper stems from the tough lower stems of the watercress; there should be about 3 packed cups. Save any remaining watercress for another use and the stems for juicing.

2. In a large saucepan, combine the watercress, onion, and rice. Add the broth and 1½ cups water. Cover and set the pot over medium-high heat. When the liquid boils, reduce the heat and simmer for 12 minutes. Remove from the heat and let the covered soup sit for 5 minutes.

3. Puree the hot soup in a super blender. Transfer the pureed soup to a heat-proof container, season with salt and pepper, cover, and refrigerate until well chilled, 4 to 24 hours.

4. To serve, adjust the seasoning and divide the cold soup among four bowls. At the table, for each serving, fill a tablespoon with cream and gently tilt it, sliding off the cream to float over the soup. Garnish with one-fourth of the chives.

To store: This soup keeps for 2 days chilled in the refrigerator.

SPINACH GAZPACHO with WALNUTS

SERVES 6 |

Inspired by Spanish white gazpacho, this cold soup is made using walnuts instead of almonds. Baby spinach and fresh herbs tint it a pale, refreshing green. Garnished with a very liberal amount of crisp raw vegetables, it entices wilted appetites on the hottest day. If you like the taste of hot chilies, toss a jalapeño into the blender along with the spinach. Using a super blender makes this soup exceptionally creamy.

1½ cups walnuts

2 garlic cloves, chopped

⅓ cup extra-virgin olive oil

3 cups ice water, divided

2 tablespoons white vinegar

1 teaspoon Sherry vinegar

2 slices white sandwich bread, torn into 1-inch pieces

2 lightly packed cups baby spinach

½ lightly packed cup flat-leaf parsley

12 basil leaves

Pinch of cayenne pepper

Salt and freshly ground pepper

FOR GARNISH

½ cup very thinly sliced Persian cucumber

½ green bell pepper, finely chopped

½ yellow bell pepper, finely chopped

½ cup very thinly sliced red radish

1 jalapeño pepper, seeded and finely chopped

1. Combine the nuts, garlic, oil, and 1 cup of the ice water in a blender, and whirl to a puree. Add the vinegars, bread, and remaining 2 cups ice water and whirl to blend in the bread. Add the spinach, parsley, basil, and cayenne and whirl to combine. Season with salt and pepper. Chill until ice cold, 4 to 24 hours.

2. To serve, recheck the seasoning, then divide the chilled soup among six bowls. Garnish with the cucumber, green and yellow bell pepper, radish, and jalapeño pepper, if using.

To store: This soup keeps for 3 days tightly covered in the refrigerator.

THE BEST VEGETABLE STOCK

MAKES 3½ QUARTS |

Vegetable stocks that look like carrot juice or reek of garlic and onions are a pet peeve of mine. Instead, this translucent liquid adds full-bodied flavor to soups, stews, and other dishes without changing their color or dominating them. It contains no added sodium, just whatever comes naturally in its abundance of vegetables. After pressing the vegetables in a strainer, if you have the patience to also squeeze them by hand, you will get an additional half-cup of stock with even more intense flavor.

2 celery ribs, with leaves, cut into 1-inch pieces

1 large carrot, diced

1 leek, white and pale green parts, chopped

1 onion, cubed

1 medium yellow-fleshed potato, diced

1 medium zucchini, coarsely chopped

½ small celery root, peeled and cubed

¼ small green cabbage, about ½ pound, coarsely chopped

¼ pound green beans, cut into 1-inch pieces

15 flat-leaf parsley sprigs

1 teaspoon whole peppercorns

1 14½-ounce can diced tomatoes

1 large bay leaf

1. In a large, nonreactive pot, combine the celery, carrot, leek, onion, potato, zucchini, celery root, cabbage, green beans, parsley, and peppercorns with 4 quarts of water. Bring to a boil over medium-high heat, reduce the heat, and simmer, uncovered, for 30 minutes.

2. Add the tomatoes with their liquid and bay leaf and simmer for 30 minutes. Let the stock cool in the pot to room temperature.

3. Set a strainer over a large bowl. Strain the stock and vegetables through the strainer into the bowl, pressing on the solids with the back of a large wooden spoon to extract as much flavor as possible. Pour the stock not being used immediately into quart jars and refrigerate. It keeps tightly covered in the refrigerator for up to 5 days. If there is sediment, give the jar a shake before using.

COOK'S TIP

Freeze the stock in resealable 1-quart plastic freezer bags and store for up to 2 months. Or freeze it in ice cube trays, then transfer the cubes to a 1-gallon plastic freezer bag and store for up to 1 month.

ALMOST HOMEMADE CHICKEN STOCK

MAKES 3¾ CUPS |

Simmering store-bought chicken stock with fresh vegetables gives it nearly made-from-scratch flavor. I use just the three basic aromatics—carrot, celery, and onion—although adding parsnip and parsley makes it even better.

1 32-ounce container fat-free reduced-sodium chicken stock, preferably organic

1 small carrot, cut into 2-inch pieces

1 small celery rib, cut into 2-inch pieces

1 large onion, quartered

2 flat-leaf parsley sprigs, or 4 plucked stems, optional

1-inch piece parsnip or celery root, optional

⅛ teaspoon peppercorns, optional

1. Combine the stock, carrot, celery, and onion in a large saucepan. If using, add the parsley, parsnip, and peppercorns. Bring the stock almost to a boil, and simmer, covered, until the vegetables are very soft, 25 minutes.

2. Set a large strainer over a bowl. Pour the stock through the strainer, pressing lightly on the vegetables with the back of a wooden spoon. Discard the solids. The enriched stock keeps tightly covered in the refrigerator for 3 days.

COOK'S TIP

Freeze unused stock in an ice cube tray. Store the cubes in a resealable plastic bag, squeezing out as much air as possible.

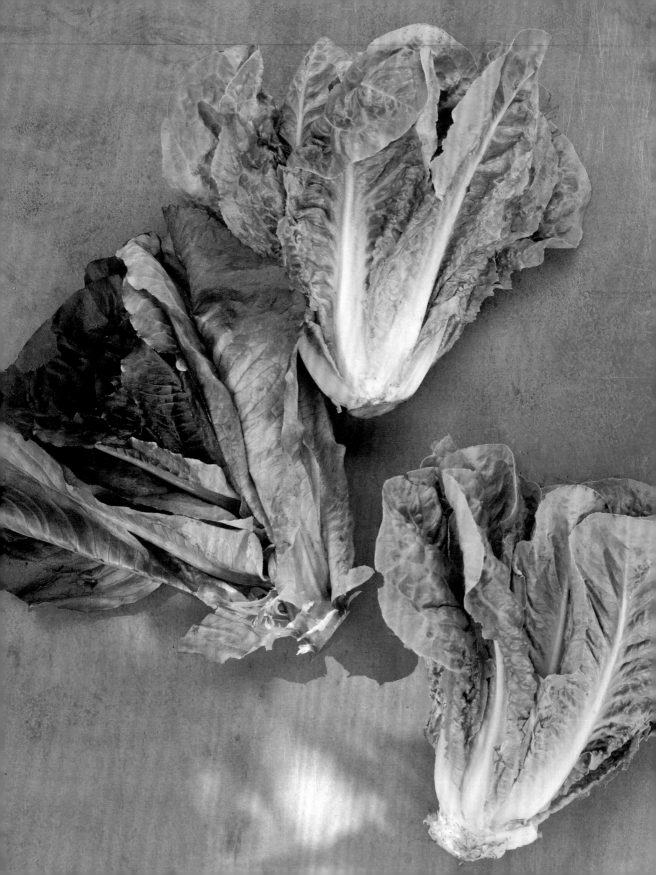

4.

SALADS

WHEN LOCAL GREENS ARE IN SEASON, MY DINNER IS often a salad of romaine lettuce topped with red radishes or sweet red peppers, plus for protein beans, hard-cooked egg, or something grilled. Living in the Northeast, the winter salads I make are noticeably different, leaning toward dark greens, which I use raw or cooked. All these salads are bold, whether they are the center of a meal or served on the side.

These nineteen salads include some that are raw, like Spicy Chopped Salad (p. 71), combining arugula, watercress, and radishes, and Caesar Salad with Parmesan Chickpeas (p. 63). The little salads that Moroccans serve inspired Beets and Beet Greens with Citrus Dressing (p. 73), an earthy combination of roasted beets and steamed greens. Using steamed vegetables with Asian flavor, there is chunky Bok Choy and Carrot Salad with Double Sesame Dressing (p. 76).

Adding whole grains is an easy way to make a salad into a main dish. Here, the grains include red quinoa, black rice, and nutty, tender farro.

I find salads that combine raw and cooked ingredients have a temperature contrast that is particularly enticing. Spinach topped with seared nectarines, and grilled romaine set on top of sun-ripe tomato slices allow either the fruit or the greens to be the warm, cooked component.

Dressings with a twist are the fun side of salads. Wasabi dressing paired with baby kale, grape tomatoes, sweet onion, and tuna (p. 85); bitters vinaigrette on asparagus, radish, and watercress salad (p. 70); and apple cider used as the dressing on turkey and kale salad with cranberries (p. 86) demonstrate this playfulness.

All these salads include high-nutrient ingredients beyond their greens. Quinoa, beans, black rice, farro, and nuts, plus citrus juices and olive oil, make them supercharged dishes for optimum health.

CAESAR SALAD with PARMESAN CHICKPEAS

SERVES 4 |

Using romaine's outer leaves and ribs gives this Caesar as much crunch as you get from the paler heart, plus the darker leaves have more nutrients. Parmesan-coated chickpeas add more crunch. They are also a good snack and garnish for soups.

PARMESAN CHICKPEAS

3 tablespoons grated Parmesan cheese

1 tablespoon extra-virgin olive oil

1 teaspoon garlic powder

½ teaspoon onion powder

½ teaspoon salt

⅛ teaspoon freshly ground pepper

1 15-ounce can chickpeas, drained

· · · · · ·

12 large romaine lettuce leaves

1 hard-cooked egg, chopped

DRESSING

2 garlic cloves, finely chopped

1 tablespoon fresh lemon juice

½ teaspoon salt

Freshly ground pepper

4 anchovy fillets, drained and chopped, optional

2 tablespoons extra-virgin olive oil

1. Preheat the oven to 400°F. Line a baking sheet with parchment paper.

2. In a medium bowl, combine the cheese, oil, garlic and onion powders, salt, and pepper to make a paste. Using paper towels, blot the chickpeas dry. Add them to the bowl, working with your fingers to coat the beans. Spread the coated chickpeas in an even layer on the prepared pan. Roast the beans for 30 minutes, stirring every 8 minutes until they are browned and hard. Cool the chickpeas to room temperature.

3. For the dressing, in a small bowl, combine the garlic, lemon juice, salt, and a generous amount of pepper. Mash in the anchovies, if using. Whisk in the oil.

4. To serve, tear the lettuce into big bite-size pieces and place them in a salad bowl. Add the dressing and toss to combine. Sprinkle on the egg and chickpeas.

A PARTY TRICK

Oil in the dressing quickly wilts salad greens. Caterers put the dressing in a deep bowl, invert a plate over it, then add the greens and refrigerate the salad for several hours. When ready to serve, they remove the plate and toss the salad.

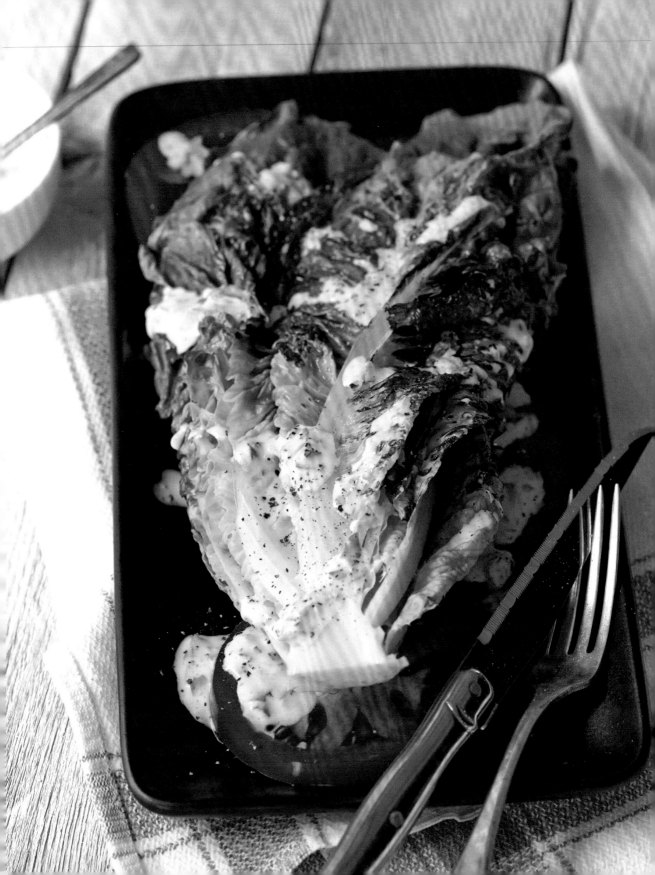

GRILLED ROMAINE LETTUCE with BEEFSTEAK TOMATOES and RANCH DRESSING

SERVES 4 |

Charring brings out the sweetness in romaine lettuce. The lightly wilted lettuce set over slabs of ripe beefsteak tomato makes a glorious summer meal. I like presenting it on an oval plate, accompanied by a serrated knife to slice into the half-head of lettuce and meaty tomatoes. A warm and cool salad, it is my favorite with steak, burgers, or grilled shrimp.

DRESSING

1 scallion, green and white parts, coarsely chopped

2 garlic cloves, coarsely chopped

¼ cup buttermilk

¼ cup sour cream

2 teaspoons rice vinegar

1 teaspoon dried oregano

1 tablespoon canola oil

1 teaspoon salt

Freshly ground pepper

・・・・・・

2 small heads red or green romaine lettuce, outer leaves removed

Extra-virgin olive oil

4 beefsteak-style tomatoes, thickly sliced

2 scallions, green part only, finely chopped

NUTRINOTE

Lettuces with red leaves or only red tips add anthocyanin benefits to salads.

---

1. Prepare a grill for direct cooking over medium-high heat or place a ridged grill pan over high heat.

2. For the dressing, in a mini food processor, pulse the scallion and garlic until finely chopped. Add the buttermilk, sour cream, vinegar, oregano, oil, salt, and a generous amount of pepper, and whirl until the dressing is well combined. Let the dressing sit for 10 minutes and up to 1 day to let the flavors develop. It keeps, covered, in the refrigerator for 3 days, thickening as it sits.

3. Halve the lettuce heads lengthwise. Trim the bases, leaving enough to hold each half together. Brush the cut side of the lettuce halves lightly with olive oil.

4. Grill the lettuce halves, cut-side down, until lightly charred, 2 to 3 minutes. Using tongs, turn the lettuce, and grill just long enough to wilt the outer leaves lightly, 1 to 2 minutes. Transfer the lettuce to four salad plates, placing it cut-side down.

5. Add 4 tomato slices to each plate, tucking them partly under the lettuce. Sprinkle on the chopped scallions and drizzle on the dressing.

SPINACH SALAD with SEARED NECTARINES and HONEY MUSTARD DRESSING

SERVES 4 |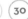

Grilled fruit goes especially well with raw spinach. Searing the fruit in a stovetop grill pan makes preparing it even easier than using an outdoor grill, plus you don't have to worry about slices landing in the fire. Serve this salad with grilled fish, pan-seared chicken cutlets, or accompanied by Spinach and Cheddar Scones (p. 200).

DRESSING

1 tablespoon fresh lemon juice

1 tablespoon red wine vinegar

1½ tablespoons wildflower honey, or 2 teaspoons dark agave syrup

1 teaspoon Dijon mustard

½ teaspoon salt

Freshly ground pepper

2 tablespoons extra-virgin olive oil

· · · · · ·

Olive oil cooking spray, or oil for brushing the nectarines

2 ripe nectarines, each cut into 8 wedges

8 lightly packed cups baby spinach

2 red onion slices

2 tablespoons sliced almonds

1. For the dressing, place the lemon juice, vinegar, honey, mustard, salt, and 3 grinds of pepper in a small jar, cover tightly, and shake to combine. Add the oil, cover, and shake vigorously. This makes about ¼ cup dressing.

2. Set a grill pan over medium-high heat until water flicked onto the pan sizzles. Spray the fingers of one hand with cooking spray and rub the nectarine wedges to coat them lightly with the oil. Grill the nectarines until they are well marked on one side, 1 to 2 minutes. Using tongs, transfer the grilled fruit to a plate, arranging the slices grilled-side up.

3. In a large bowl, toss the spinach with the dressing, coating it lightly. Divide the spinach among four salad plates. Separate the onion slices into rings and arrange them on top of the spinach. Add 4 nectarine wedges to each plate, placing them grilled-side up. Sprinkle on the sliced almonds. Serve immediately.

To store: Leftover dressing keeps tightly covered in the refrigerator for 1 day. Combine it with some shredded cabbage and carrot for coleslaw.

COOK'S TIP

Grilling the nectarines on just one side keeps them pleasantly firm while adding smoky flavor and caramelizing the fruit nicely.

ARUGULA, ENDIVE, and AVOCADO SALAD with MEYER LEMON VINAIGRETTE

SERVES 4 |

Think about serving this composed salad of bitter greens and luxurious avocado as the first course at dinner parties or with a casual pizza dinner. For the dressing, if Meyer lemons are unavailable, use a combination of fresh-squeezed lemon and orange juice.

4 lightly packed cups baby arugula

1 medium endive (5 to 6 ounces), cut crosswise into ½-inch slices

4 thin red onion slices

DRESSING

4 teaspoons Meyer lemon juice

½ teaspoon salt

Freshly ground pepper

2 tablespoons mild extra-virgin olive oil, such as Kirkland organic or Zoë

· · · · · ·

1 ripe Hass avocado, halved, pitted, and peeled

1. In a mixing bowl, combine the arugula, endive, and onion, separating the onion into rings.

2. In a small bowl, whisk the lemon juice and salt together until the salt dissolves, 1 minute. Add 3 or 4 grinds of pepper. Whisk in the oil. Use two forks to toss the salad with the dressing just until the salad glistens. Divide the dressed salad among four salad plates.

3. Cut the avocado lengthwise into 12 slices. Peel and arrange 3 slices in a fan on top of each salad. Serve immediately.

COOK'S TIP

To make this salad ahead of time without the avocado discoloring, lay the slices out on a plate and brush lightly with oil. Cover the plate with plastic wrap, pressing it against the avocado, and refrigerate for up to 4 hours. The greens and dressing, covered with plastic wrap and refrigerated, keep for 4 hours, too.

TUSCAN KALE SALAD with POMEGRANATE SEEDS and WALNUTS

SERVES 4 |

Tart-sweet pomegranate, walnuts, and cilantro balance the bitter side of kale nicely. Protein in the kale and nuts means this salad can stand alone as well as accompany a sandwich or cooked chops.

1 cup pomegranate juice

1 medium bunch Tuscan kale (12 ounces), stemmed and finely shredded, 5 to 6 cups

1 tablespoon extra-virgin olive oil

½ teaspoon salt

¾ cup fresh pomegranate seeds

¾ cup walnuts, chopped

3 tablespoons finely chopped red onion

Freshly ground pepper

⅓ cup chopped cilantro

1. In a small saucepan, boil the pomegranate juice until it is reduced to ¼ cup, 15 to 18 minutes. Set aside to cool.

2. In a large mixing bowl, massage the kale with the oil and salt until wilted, 1 minute. Set it aside for 30 minutes.

3. Toss the pomegranate seeds, walnuts, and onion with the wilted kale. Add 3 tablespoons of the reduced pomegranate juice, season with pepper, and toss.

4. Just before serving, mix in the cilantro.

To store: The prepared salad keeps covered in the refrigerator for 4 days.

THE BEST WAY TO SEED A POMEGRANATE

Wear an apron to avoid permanent pink polka dots on your clothes. Work in the sink to minimize juice spattering on the walls, too.

Cut off the topknot, then score the pomegranate's skin in quarters, like a navel orange. Cradle the fruit in your hands over a bowl, press both thumbs into the top of the pomegranate, and pull it into two halves. Break the halves in two. Pull away the pale, papery membrane covering the seeds and with your fingertips tickle out the seeds.

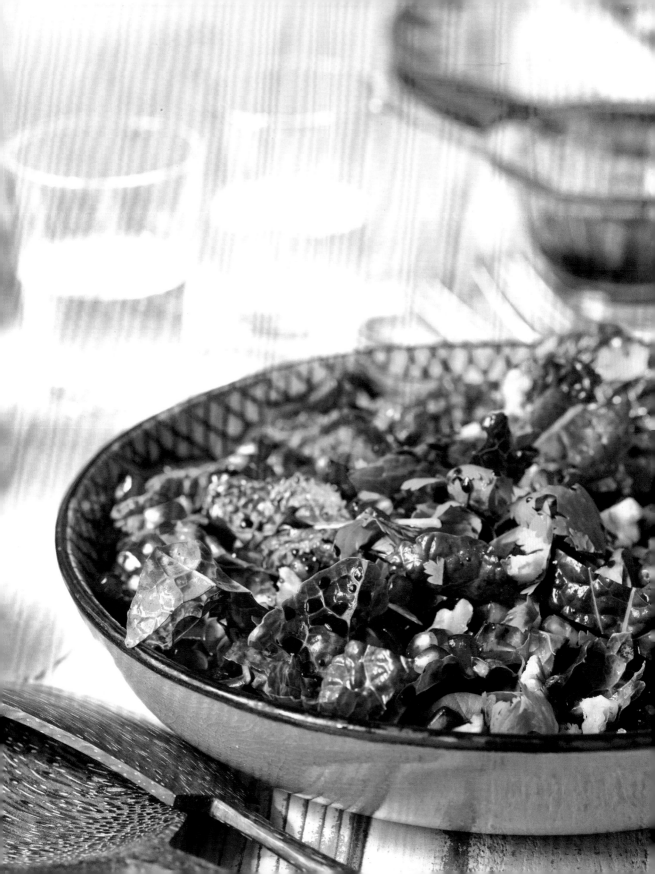

ASPARAGUS, RADISH, and WATERCRESS SALAD with BITTERS VINAIGRETTE

SERVES 4 |

Pairing bitters with watercress and radishes, which also taste bitter, seems counterintuitive but they play together nicely. To make this composed salad a colorful centerpiece for a buffet, present it on a big platter, family style. Serve it along with grilled salmon, Tofu Piccata (p. 102), or pizza.

½ pound asparagus, stems trimmed, cut into 1-inch pieces

2 teaspoon fresh lemon juice

1 teaspoon champagne vinegar

4 drops Angostura bitters

½ teaspoon salt

Freshly ground pepper

4 teaspoons extra-virgin olive oil

2 cups baby arugula

½ bunch watercress, coarse stems removed

4 large radishes, thinly sliced

4 teaspoons snipped chives

1. In a large saucepan fitted with a steamer insert, steam the asparagus for 1 minute. Using tongs, transfer the asparagus to a large bowl. Immediately cool the asparagus under cold running water. Drain the asparagus well.

2. In a large salad bowl or mixing bowl, combine the lemon juice, vinegar, bitters, salt, and 3 or 4 grinds of pepper. Whisk to dissolve the salt, then whisk in the oil. Gently place the arugula and cress in the salad bowl on top of the dressing, then arrange the radishes and asparagus over the greens. At this point, the salad can be covered with plastic wrap and refrigerated for up to 2 hours before serving.

3. To serve, use two forks to toss the salad with the dressing, then divide it among four salad plates. Sprinkle one-fourth of the chives over each serving. Serve immediately.

ANOTHER WAY

For a party, arrange the arugula and watercress in a ring around the outside of a large platter. In a bowl, dress the asparagus and radishes, then arrange them in the center of the plate. Drizzle the remaining dressing in the bowl over the greens.

SPICY CHOPPED SALAD

SERVES 4 |

Every Mediterranean restaurant, falafel stand, and hummus bar serves a chopped salad made with cucumber, tomato, onion, and scallion. Often it's as flavorful as iceberg lettuce. To make one with *taïm* (Hebrew for "taste"), I add arugula and watercress and replace the usually unripe tomato with red radish. Toss this chunky salad with a puckery citrus dressing and serve it as part of a meze spread including Roasted Red Peppers Stuffed with Kale (p. 31) and Collard Green Dolmas (p. 33), or add feta cheese and store-bought stuffed grape leaves to turn this salad into a main dish.

2 lightly packed cups baby arugula

1 lightly packed cup watercress sprigs

1 large Persian cucumber, peeled and sliced, or 6-inch European cucumber, peeled, seeded, and chopped

1 medium red bell pepper, seeded and chopped

4 large red radishes, sliced and quartered

1 large scallion, white and green parts, chopped

DRESSING

1 tablespoon fresh lemon juice

1 tablespoon white wine vinegar

1 teaspoon salt

Freshly ground pepper

2 teaspoons raw agave syrup

2 tablespoons extra-virgin olive oil

1. Coarsely chop the arugula and watercress and place them in a mixing bowl. Add the cucumber, red pepper, radishes, and scallion, using two forks to toss and combine the salad.

2. For the dressing, in a small bowl, whisk the lemon juice and vinegar with the salt and 3 or 4 grinds of pepper until the salt dissolves. Mix in the agave until blended. Whisk in the oil. Or, you can store the dressing and undressed salad separately in the refrigerator for 8 hours before combining them.

3. To serve, dress and toss the salad. Divide it among four salad plates.

NUTRINOTE

Radishes, a cruciferous vegetable, get their heat from health-protecting sulfur compounds.

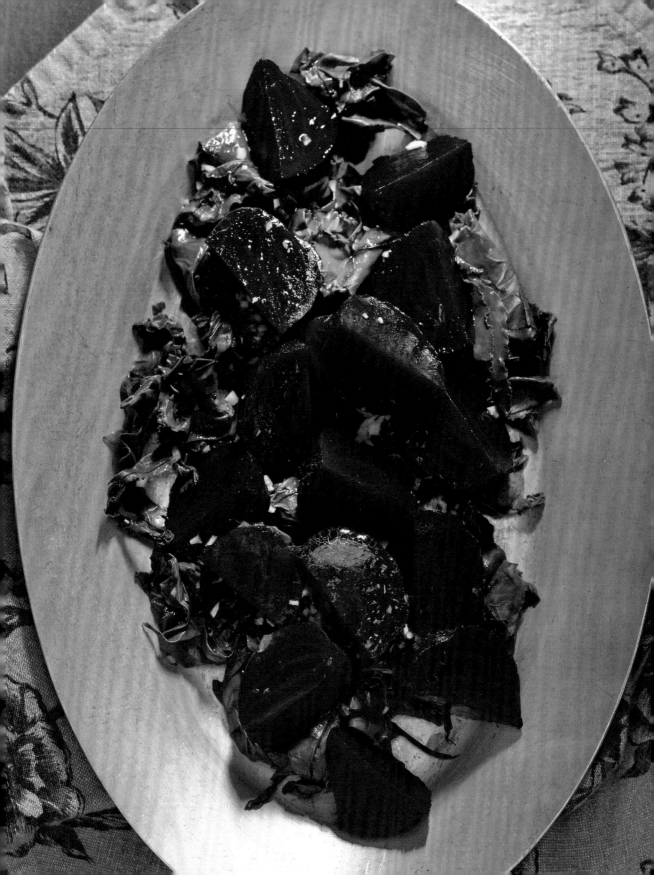

BEETS and BEET GREENS with CITRUS DRESSING

SERVES 4 |

For me, a bunch of beets is a two-fer, like the bonus of getting two Broadway theater tickets for the price of one. Along with sweet, earthy beets, you also get their greens, which taste like a cross between spinach and red chard. Served together and bathed in a ginger dressing, they are always a hit. Serve with sliced grilled steak, or make a vegetarian plate together with cooked beans and quinoa.

½ small garlic clove, finely chopped

1 inch fresh ginger, peeled and chopped

2 tablespoons orange juice

½ teaspoon fresh lemon juice, optional

½ teaspoon salt

Freshly ground pepper

1 tablespoon extra-virgin olive oil

4 medium red beets

Greens from 1 large or 2 medium bunches of beets

1. Place the garlic, ginger, orange juice, lemon juice if using, salt, and 3 or 4 grinds of pepper in a small jar. Cover and shake the jar. Add the oil and set the jar aside to let the flavors develop and blend.

2. In a deep saucepan, cover the beets with cold water to a depth of 2 inches and cook over medium-high heat, partially covered, until a small knife easily pierces them. Transfer the beets to a plate until they are cool enough to handle. Leave 1 inch of water in the pot.

3. Cut the stems off at the bases of the beet leaves or fold the front sides together like closing a book, and pull the leaf away from the stem and center vein. Discard the stems and veins. Wash the leaves in a large bowl of cold water, paying particular attention to the crevices where sand hides, and changing the water several times. Coarsely chop the leaves; there should be about 6 packed cups.

4. Add the chopped beet greens to the pot with the reserved cooking water, and bring to a boil. Using a wooden spoon, push the greens into the water and cook until almost tender, 5 to 6 minutes. Drain the beet greens in a colander, and set aside until cool enough to handle.

5. To avoid staining your hands, slip them into sandwich-size plastic bags and peel the beets. Cut them into ½-inch slices. Arrange the sliced beets in an overlapping ring around the edge of a serving plate.

continued on next page

6. Squeeze the excess moisture out of the cooled greens, pull apart the compressed leaves, and mound them in the center of the plate. You can cover the arranged salad with plastic wrap and refrigerate it for 8 hours. Store the dressing separately.

7. To serve, shake the dressing vigorously for 15 seconds, then strain it over the beets and greens.

ANOTHER WAY

Beet greens are also good simply drizzled with good-quality olive oil and a spritz of fresh lemon juice.

ASK THE FARMER

Shoppers at farm stands often have the farmer tear the tops off their bunch of beets. Ask for any extra greens when you purchase your beets.

BRUSSELS SPROUTS and BROCCOLI LEAF SLAW

SERVES 8 |

Fans of kale salad love this combination inspired by a cabbage and kale slaw I found at a deli in a Polish neighborhood in Brooklyn, N.Y. Super-crunchy when freshly made, this salad gets more supple as it sits. Serve it with sausages or grilled veggie burgers, including Black Bean and Broccoli Leaf Burgers (p. 196).

7 broccoli leaves (about ½ bunch), center veins and stems removed

1 pound Brussels sprouts

1 large carrot, coarsely shredded

1 cup chopped scallions, green part only

DRESSING

2 tablespoons white vinegar

1 tablespoon sugar

1 teaspoon salt

Freshly ground pepper

1 tablespoon cold-pressed coconut oil

1. Separate the stripped broccoli leaves lengthwise into two halves. Stack 3 or 4 halves and roll them into a long, loose cigar. Cut the leaves crosswise into very thin strips, making about 3½ cups finely shredded broccoli leaf. Place the shredded leaves in a large mixing bowl.

2. Cut the Brussels sprouts crosswise into thin slices. While adding them to the broccoli leaf, pull the sliced Brussels sprouts apart into shreds. Add the carrot and scallions to the bowl, and toss with your hands to combine them with the broccoli leaves and Brussels sprouts.

3. For the dressing, in a small bowl, whisk the vinegar, sugar, and salt together until the sugar dissolves. Add 5 or 6 grinds of pepper. Whisk in the oil and pour the dressing over the shredded vegetables. Massage the salad with your fingers until the broccoli leaves and Brussels sprouts have softened, 2 minutes. Cover the bowl with plastic wrap and refrigerate the slaw for at least 1 hour or up to 24 hours before serving.

To store: This slaw keeps tightly covered in the refrigerator for up to 4 days.

NUTRINOTE

A serving of these greens provides 4 grams of protein, as much as an egg white.

BOK CHOY and CARROT SALAD with DOUBLE SESAME DRESSING

SERVES 4 |

This chunky salad has the crispness of lightly pickled Asian vegetables. Steaming helps the vegetables absorb the dressing and also lets your body better use their nutrients. Serve this salad alongside grilled chicken, pork, or tofu dishes.

2 teaspoons sesame seeds

2 medium carrots

1 small head bok choy (8 ounces), or 3 stalks from a large head

2 tablespoons orange juice

1 teaspoon rice vinegar

¼ teaspoon reduced-sodium soy sauce

¼ teaspoon grated ginger

½ teaspoon sugar

½ teaspoon salt

1 teaspoon toasted sesame oil

1. In a small skillet over medium-high heat, toast the sesame seeds, shaking the pan until the seeds are lightly colored and fragrant, 4 minutes. Cool the sesame seeds on a plate.

2. Cut the carrots diagonally into ½-inch slices. Cut the white part of the bok choy into ½-inch slices. Slice the green part of one leaf into fine strips. Use the remaining bok choy leaves in a stir-fry or juice.

3. In a pot fitted with a steamer insert, steam the carrots until crisp-tender, 4 minutes. Transfer them to a colander and cool under cold running water. Steam the bok choy for 1 minute, add to the carrots, and cool. Spin-dry the vegetables and place them in a medium bowl.

4. For the dressing, in a small bowl, whisk together the orange juice, vinegar, soy sauce, ginger, sugar, and salt until the sugar dissolves. Whisk in the sesame oil and half the sesame seeds.

5. To serve, toss the carrots and bok choy with the dressing. Sprinkle on the shredded bok choy leaf and remaining sesame seeds.

COOK'S TIP

A sprinkling of finely shredded raw bok choy leaves makes a nice garnish on cooked rice.

RED QUINOA TABBOULEH

SERVES 4 |

I make tabbouleh using lots of vegetables. I prefer using gluten-free quinoa instead of bulgur because it feels easier to digest. Red quinoa is especially good in this oil-free salad, which is even better after it marinates in its lemon juice dressing overnight. Serve with Roasted Red Peppers Stuffed with Kale (p. 31) or store-bought falafel.

1 medium red bell pepper, seeded and finely chopped

1 small zucchini squash, about 5 inches, halved lengthwise, seeded, and finely chopped

½ cup chopped cilantro

½ cup chopped flat-leaf parsley

½ cup finely chopped scallions, green part only

¾ cup cooked red quinoa, prepared according to package directions

2 tablespoons fresh lemon juice

½ teaspoon salt

Freshly ground pepper

⅓ cup snipped fresh dill

1. Place the red pepper, zucchini, cilantro, parsley, scallions, and quinoa in a mixing bowl and use a fork to combine them.

2. In a small bowl, whisk the lemon juice, salt, and 4 or 5 grinds of the pepper together until the salt dissolves. Pour the dressing over the tabbouleh and toss to combine. Mix in the dill. Cover with plastic wrap and refrigerate the tabbouleh for 1 to 24 hours before serving. This salad keeps tightly covered in the refrigerator for 2 days.

ANOTHER WAY

Scoop some tabbouleh into a pita bread lined with shredded romaine lettuce and add crumbled feta cheese for a light meal.

ENDIVE, WATERCRESS, and PEAR SALAD

SERVES 4 |

Serving watercress and endive used to show you were sophisticated and well-heeled. Now it says you are smart and health-conscious. Functionally, their bitterness stimulates the appetite and digestion, precisely what a salad should do. Ripe pear and blue cheese add elegance, making this salad the perfect first course at a dinner party. Follow it with pork tenderloin, filet of beef, or Salmon Steamed in a Cabbage Leaf with Corn Butter (p. 105). To serve it casually, make a bed of the watercress, lay whole endive leaves and pear wedges on top of it, sprinkle on the cheese and nuts, and serve with an omelet or quiche. Replace the walnut oil with all canola or grapeseed oil, if you prefer.

DRESSING

1 tablespoon white wine vinegar

½ teaspoon salt

Freshly ground pepper

2 tablespoons Dijon mustard

2 tablespoons roasted walnut oil

2 tablespoons canola or grapeseed oil

. . . . . .

2 medium heads endive, 5 to 6 ounces each

1 large Bartlett pear

1 bunch watercress

4 tablespoons (2 ounces) crumbled Roquefort or other blue cheese, optional

2 tablespoons walnuts, optional, for garnish

1. For the dressing, in a small bowl, combine the vinegar, salt, and 4 or 5 grinds of pepper. Whisk in the mustard. While whisking, slowly drizzle in the walnut and canola oils.

2. Cut the endive crosswise into 1-inch rounds. Over a mixing bowl, separate the slices into leafy strips, discarding any hard core. Slice the pear lengthwise into quarters. Core each quarter, cut it into 5 long slices, and add the pear to the endive. Pluck the leafy sprigs off the tougher watercress stems and add them to the endive and pear, tossing gently with your hands to combine them.

3. Divide the salad among four plates, arranging it to show the colorful pear skin as much as possible. Using a tablespoon, drizzle one-fourth of the dressing over each salad. Sprinkle on the cheese and/or toasted walnuts.

GOOD TECHNIQUE

To toast walnuts, preheat the oven to 350°F. Spread the chopped nuts on a small baking sheet. Bake for 5 minutes. Stir and bake for 3 minutes longer, or until the walnuts are fragrant and lightly colored. Transfer the nuts to a plate to cool.

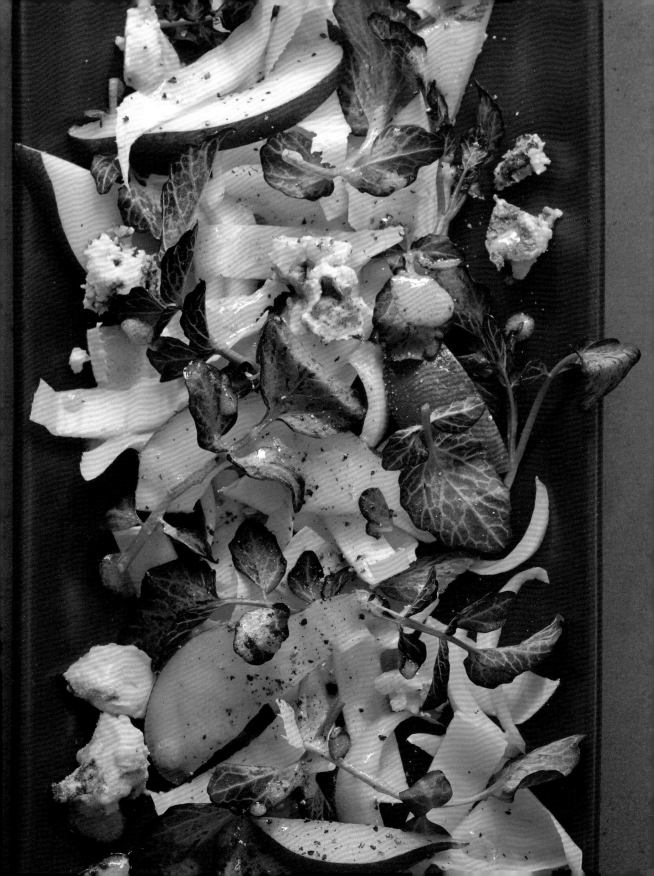

POTATO SALAD with GREEN PEAS and WATERCRESS

SERVES 4 |

The Japanese use fiery wasabi root in mashed potatoes that are amazing. Blending it into a creamy dressing has the same surprising, irresistible effect. The potatoes soak up the dressing quickly, so add it shortly before serving. Potatoes small enough to eat in one or two bites are fun to use. Since you eat the skin, I prefer using organic potatoes.

DRESSING

¼ cup sour cream, full fat or reduced fat

¼ cup buttermilk, full fat or light

1 tablespoon fresh lemon juice

1 tablespoon red wine vinegar

1 teaspoon wasabi paste

1 teaspoon olive oil

Salt and freshly ground pepper

· · · · · ·

1¼ pounds small red-skinned new potatoes, preferably organic

½ cup frozen baby green peas, defrosted

2 tablespoons finely chopped shallots

½ cup tender watercress sprigs

¼ cup snipped fresh dill

1. In a small bowl, combine the sour cream, buttermilk, lemon juice, vinegar, and wasabi. Whisk in the oil and season with salt and pepper. Set the dressing aside.

2. In a large saucepan, cover the potatoes with cold water by 2 inches. Bring to a boil over high heat, reduce the heat, and cook, uncovered, until the potatoes are tender when pierced with a knife, about 15 minutes from when the water boils. Drain the potatoes and place them in a medium bowl. If the potatoes are 1½ inches or larger, when cool enough to handle, halve or quarter them.

3. Add the peas and shallots to the warm potatoes. At this point, the salad can sit at room temperature for up to 1 hour.

4. Pour the dressing over the potato salad, and toss to blend. Add the watercress and dill and toss. Adjust the seasonings, and serve, preferably within 1 hour of adding the dressing. This salad is best served the day it is made but leftovers keep tightly covered in the refrigerator for 24 hours.

NUTRINOTE

To cut calories, you can use reduced-fat sour cream and buttermilk. Avoid the fat-free versions, which will make your salad taste pasty.

ABOUT WASABI

Wasabi paste sold in a tube keeps for about a year because it contains preservatives. I prefer using the canned powder, making sure that the ingredients list wasabi ahead of mustard powder or horseradish. Both are added because wasabi is expensive and they provide filler that helps to keep the cost down.

BLACK RICE SALAD with RED CHARD and CRANBERRIES

SERVES 4 |

I first served this as a hot side dish. Then I ate it as leftovers and it was even better. A smart cook surrenders to the unexpected, so here it is as a grain-based salad substantial enough to even be a main dish. Together the chard, rice, and cranberries provide enough contrast and moisture that no dressing is needed. Serve with Mulligatawny Soup with Mustard Greens (p. 50), or with cooked beans and a fresh green salad for a complete meatless meal.

⅓ cup black rice, preferably Lotus Foods Forbidden Rice (see Note)

3 large red chard leaves or 5 medium leaves, center veins and stems removed

1 tablespoon extra-virgin olive oil

1 large shallot, chopped

⅓ cup dried cranberries

¼ teaspoon ground allspice

Salt and freshly ground pepper

1. In a medium saucepan, combine the rice with 1¼ cups water and cook, covered, until the rice is tender but not soft, about 20 minutes. Let the rice rest, covered, for 10 minutes. Uncover and let the rice cool.

2. Meanwhile, in a covered, large saucepan, boil 4 cups of water over high heat. Add the chard, using a wooden spoon to push the leaves into the water until they collapse. Cook, covered, for 3 minutes over medium-high heat. Drain in a colander, then run cold water over the chard while swishing with your hand until it feels cool, 30 seconds. Lift the chard and press it gently to extract the excess water. Finely chop the compacted chard. Squeeze the chopped chard again and pull it apart; there will be about 1 cup.

3. In a medium skillet, heat the oil over medium-high heat. Cook the shallot, stirring often, until it softens, 4 minutes. Remove from the heat and add the chard, rice, cranberries, and allspice, and mix to combine them. Season the salad with salt and pepper. This salad is best served the day you make it.

COOK'S TIP

Forbidden Rice from Lotus Foods has the fullest flavor and it is less starchy than other brands of black rice.

FARRO SALAD with FETA and GREEN OLIVES

SERVES 4 |

Italian farro swells as it cooks, becoming fluffy and light. Green olives and feta cheese are pleasingly tangy against the sweetly nutty taste of this tender grain, an unhybridized ancient form of wheat. Serve spooned into whole romaine lettuce leaves, or together with Roasted Red Peppers Stuffed with Kale (p. 31) for an adventurous Mediterranean lunch.

¾ cup farro

4 pitted Sicilian-style olives, coarsely chopped

⅓ cup (3½ ounces) crumbled feta cheese

¼ cup chopped marinated sun-dried tomatoes

1½ teaspoons dried oregano

Freshly ground pepper

1 tablespoon red wine vinegar

1 tablespoon extra-virgin olive oil, preferably full-flavored

½ cup chopped flat-leaf parsley

Romaine lettuce and fresh mint leaves, for garnish

1. In a medium saucepan, combine the farro and 2½ cups water. Cover and bring to a boil over medium-high heat. Reduce the heat and simmer until the farro is tender, about 20 minutes. Transfer the farro to a mixing bowl and cool to room temperature.

2. Add the olives, feta, sun-dried tomatoes, oregano, and 5 or 6 grinds pepper, tossing with a fork to combine them with the farro. Add the vinegar and oil, and mix. Mix in the parsley.

3. To serve, line a platter with shredded romaine lettuce. Mound the salad on top of the lettuce and garnish with sliced mint leaves.

To store: Cooked farro turns hard when refrigerated, so serve this salad the day it is made.

NUTRINOTE

Some gluten-sensitive people tolerate farro, which is related to spelt, another variety of unhybridized wheat.

CHICKEN SALAD with BABY BOK CHOY and BROCCOLI

SERVES 4 | GF 30

The inspiration for this salad is the Chinese chicken salad that originated in San Francisco's Chinatown in the 1950s. Created for American diners, it combined chicken and canned mandarin oranges with chow mein noodles and soy dressing. This updated version calls for roast chicken—store-bought or homemade leftovers—broccoli, plus raw bok choy, a crisp apple in place of the noodles, and the brightness of fresh clementines. The dressing is a French-style vinaigrette with Asian flavors. It can be made ahead and held without refrigerating.

2 cups small broccoli florets

2 cups baby bok choy, cut crosswise into ¾-inch pieces

½ Fuji apple, peeled, cored, and diced

1 clementine, peeled and cut crosswise into rounds

1 cup roasted chicken breast (4 ounces), cubed

3 tablespoons sliced almonds, toasted

1 medium shallot, thinly sliced crosswise

DRESSING

1 teaspoon fresh lemon juice

1 teaspoon rice vinegar

⅛ teaspoon fish sauce

½ teaspoon Dijon mustard

Freshly ground pepper

2 tablespoons canola oil

Salt

1. In a large saucepan of boiling water, cook the broccoli for 3 minutes. Drain in a colander, then transfer the broccoli to a large bowl and cool under cold running water. Drain well and place the broccoli in a mixing bowl.

2. Add the bok choy and apple to the broccoli. Pull apart the clementine rounds into individual little wedges and add them to the bowl. Mix in the chicken, almonds, and shallot, separated into rings. The acid in the clementine will keep the apple from turning brown, so you can cover and refrigerate the assembled salad for up to 4 hours.

3. For the dressing, in a small bowl, whisk together the lemon juice, vinegar, fish sauce, mustard, and 4 or 5 grinds of pepper. Whisk in the oil. Season the dressing to taste with salt. Pour the dressing over the salad, using two forks to gently toss it. Divide the salad among four wide, shallow salad bowls and serve.

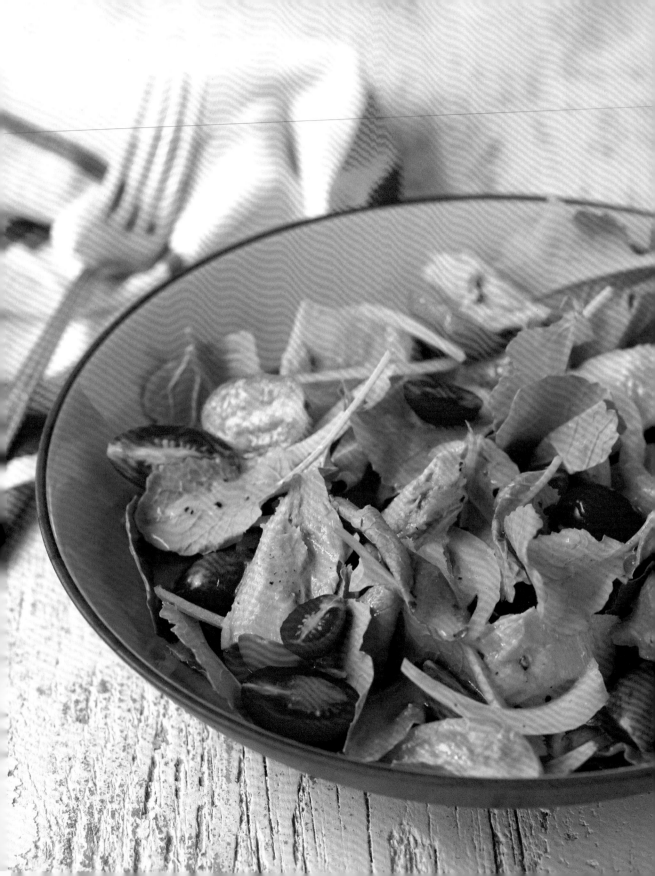

BABY KALE and TUNA SALAD with GRAPE TOMATOES, SWEET ONION, and WASABI DRESSING

SERVES 2 |

The head-clearing kick of wasabi is a fun surprise in this chunky tuna salad. Of course, wasabi goes well with tuna but it is good with the tomatoes and kale, too. Any kind of baby kale—green, red, or mixed—will work.

1 teaspoon wasabi paste or powder

1 tablespoon fresh lemon juice

¾ teaspoon salt

Freshly ground pepper

1 tablespoon fruity extra-virgin olive oil

4 packed cups baby kale leaves

1 cup grape tomatoes, halved lengthwise

½ cup sweet onion, in thin crescents

1 can water-packed tongol tuna, drained

1. In a small bowl, whisk the wasabi with the lemon juice; if using wasabi powder, also mix in 1 teaspoon water, and set aside for 10 minutes to let the heat develop. Mix in the salt, and 4 or 5 grinds of pepper, then whisk in the oil. Set the dressing aside for the flavors to meld while you make the salad.

2. Arrange the kale to cover a small platter. Sprinkle the tomatoes and onion over the greens. Add the tuna, breaking it into chunks or coarse flakes. Just before serving, pour the dressing over the salad and toss to combine.

NUTRINOTE

Tongol tuna is the canned tuna lowest in mercury and a good source of omega-3 fatty acids.

TURKEY and KALE SALAD with CRANBERRIES and CIDER DRESSING

SERVES 4 |

To make this a main dish, I thought of how well kale goes with turkey, cranberries, and an apple. A kiwifruit and curry powder bring juicy tartness and spicy warmth that make this salad stand out. Since massaging coats the kale with oil, using the flavored cider left over from plumping the cranberries works nicely as the dressing.

½ cup dried cranberries

⅓ cup apple cider

1 medium bunch (12 ounces) Tuscan kale, center veins and stems removed

1 tablespoon hemp, walnut, or canola oil

1 teaspoon salt

6 ounces roast turkey breast, diced

1 medium Granny Smith apple, peeled, cored, and diced

1 kiwi, peeled and diced

¼ teaspoon curry powder

Freshly ground pepper

1. In a small bowl, plump the cranberries in the cider, about 20 minutes.

2. Two or three leaves at a time, stack the kale and cut the leaves crosswise into fine strips, ⅜ to ½ inch. Place the kale in a medium mixing bowl, and add the oil plus ½ teaspoon salt. With your fingertips, massage the kale until it is soft; the amount of time required depends on how tender the leaves are, but 3 to 5 minutes is usually good.

3. Add the turkey, apple, and kiwi to the kale. Drain the cranberries, reserving the cider. Add the cranberries to the kale. In a small bowl, mix 3 tablespoons of the cider with the curry powder, ½ teaspoon salt, and 4 grinds of pepper. Pour this over the kale and, using a fork, mix to combine the salad. This salad can be refrigerated, covered, for up to 4 hours before serving.

4. To serve, divide the salad among four wide, shallow bowls. This salad keeps tightly covered in the refrigerator for 1 day.

BANGKOK BEEF SALAD

SERVES 4 | GF

I love how Thai cooks use aromatic fresh herbs abundantly. Here, cilantro and mint are as much the body of this salad as watercress and its other vegetables. A health-conscious carnivore, I like how their lightness balances the meat. It is okay to combine the greens ahead of time but they collapse quickly and drastically when the dressing is added, so serve the completed salad immediately.

2 garlic cloves, sliced

2 tablespoons fish sauce

1½ tablespoons fresh lime juice

2 teaspoons grated ginger

1 tablespoon canola oil

. . . . . .

1 16-ounce flank steak

5 inches European cucumber, halved lengthwise, seeded, and thinly sliced

3 large red radishes, thinly sliced

2 packed cups watercress sprigs, 1 (4-ounce) bag or 1 medium bunch

½ cup lightly packed cilantro sprigs

½ cup lightly packed mint leaves

½ medium red onion, cut into thin crescents

1 long red chile pepper, thinly sliced, seed optional

4 to 6 large basil leaves

. . . . . .

1 tablespoon raw agave syrup

½ teaspoon red Thai chili paste

Freshly ground pepper

1. For the marinade, in a small bowl, combine the garlic, fish sauce, lime juice, ginger, and oil. Pour half the marinade into a one-gallon resealable plastic bag, including all the garlic. Add the flank steak and seal the bag, pressing out all the air. Marinate the meat in the refrigerator for 2 to 4 hours, turning the bag over two or three times.

2. Prepare a grill for cooking over high heat. Pat the meat dry and grill it for 5 minutes on each side for medium rare, or longer, to your taste. Set the meat aside on a plate for 10 minutes to rest. Discard the marinade.

3. While the meat rests, in a large bowl, combine the cucumber, radishes, watercress, cilantro, mint, onion, and sliced chile pepper. Stack the basil leaves, roll them into a long tube, cut the basil crosswise into ¼-inch slivers, and add them to the bowl with the salad.

4. Cut the steak crosswise into thin slices. Cut the slices crosswise into 2-inch pieces. Add the beef to the bowl with the salad. Whisk the agave, Thai chili paste, and 6 to 8 grinds of pepper into the reserved marinade. Add the dressing to the salad and toss to combine. Serve immediately.

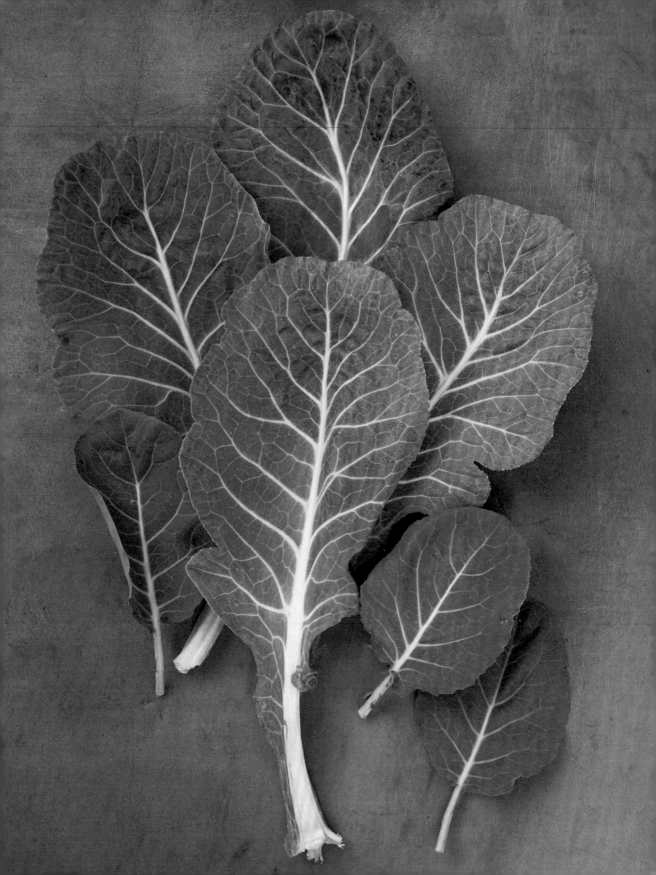

5.
MAIN DISHES

FRIENDS TEASE ME ABOUT BEING ADDICTED TO GREENS. Maybe it's true since I eat them every day. On busy days, this may simply be chard mixed into a pot of lentils. Or I put a pan-seared chicken cutlet on top of a bed of arugula. Since I include protein at most meals, when planning the main dish of the day, I often think about how to pair it with greens.

Pairing Power Greens and protein in ways that feel natural at the center of the plate is easy when there are so many of both to choose from. I use thirteen kinds of greens in these main dishes, and chicken, beans, tofu, fish, meat, lentils, cheese, eggs, or grains, plus nuts, to provide the protein. Many of the dishes are meatless, from Creole-style beans simmered with collard greens to grilled eggplant with a vegan arugula pesto.

Greening a beef stir-fry with bok choy is a no-brainer. Greek Lentil Stew (p. 95) seasoned with warm cinnamon and oregano and Turkey Hash with Sweet Potatoes and Greens (p. 110) show how chard fits into main dishes.

Then there are unexpected combinations, including Pomegranate Shrimp Curry (p. 99) liberally showered with cilantro, Salmon Steamed in a Cabbage Leaf with Corn Butter (p. 105), and cod roasted with ratatouille made with chard stems. Finally, if you like pork, "Porchetta" Roast Pork Loin Stuffed with Broccoli Rabe (p. 119) is a dish friends will talk about again and again.

The best thing about all these dishes, along with their bold flavors, is the amount of protein and the servings of greens you get.

RED BEANS and SMOKY GREENS

SERVES 4 |

Rather than cooking up a mess of greens and making a separate pot of beans, cooking them together lets the juices from the greens mingle deliciously with the beans. Here, green bell pepper, celery, and onion, the trinity of Creole cooking, add Louisiana savor while Spanish pimenton in place of andouille sausage, smoked turkey, or ham hock adds smoky depth to this vegan dish. Serve with Incendiary Herbed Brown Rice (p. 137), or Brussels Sprouts and Broccoli Leaf Slaw (p. 75).

1 medium bunch collard greens (10 to 12 ounces), center veins and stems removed, cut into 3/4-inch strips

1 tablespoon canola oil

1 medium onion, chopped

1 large celery rib, chopped

1 small green bell pepper, seeded and chopped

1 small red bell pepper, seeded and chopped

2 cloves garlic, minced

1 14-ounce can diced tomatoes, preferably roasted

1 15-ounce can red kidney beans, drained

1/2 teaspoon smoked paprika

2 teaspoons dried thyme

Salt and freshly ground pepper

1. In a covered, large saucepan, boil 6 cups of water over high heat. Add the collard greens, pushing them into the water with a wooden spoon. Cook until they are tender, 5 minutes. Drain the collard greens in a colander, then run cold water over them while swishing with your hand until they feel cool, 30 seconds. Squeeze the collards to remove excess water. Chop the collards, then pull them apart; there will be about 1 cup.

2. In a small Dutch oven or heavy, large saucepan, heat the oil over medium-high heat. Add the onion and celery and cook, stirring often, until the onion is translucent, 4 minutes. Cover, reduce the heat to medium-low, and cook for 10 minutes to draw the juices from the vegetables and concentrate them.

3. Raise the heat to medium-high. Mix in the peppers and garlic, and cook, stirring occasionally, until the vegetables are almost dry, 3 to 4 minutes.

4. Add the tomatoes with their liquid, the beans, collard greens, paprika, and thyme. Pour in 3 cups water. Bring the liquid to a boil, reduce the heat to medium-low, and simmer, uncovered, until the greens are tender, about 15 minutes. Season with salt and pepper.

To store: This dish keeps tightly covered in the refrigerator for 4 days. Reheat it in a covered heavy saucepan over medium-high heat, stirring occasionally, adding 1/2 cup of vegetable broth or water, if needed.

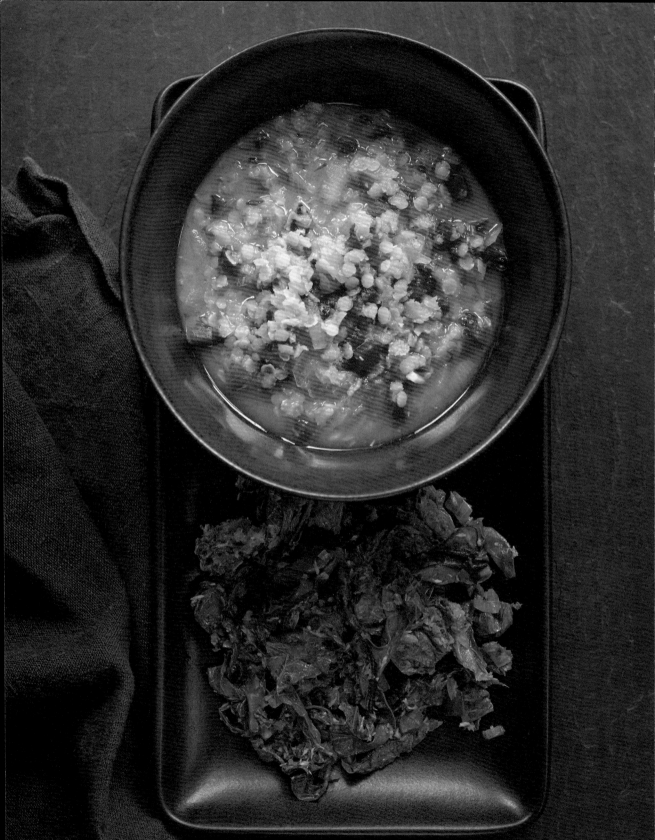

INDIAN GREENS with LEMON DAL

SERVES 4 |

Slightly soupy dal made from lentils or other legumes is a main source of protein for many Indians. They eat dal every day, using it as a dip, a sauce, or a side dish. Here red lentils are simmered with garlic and rosemary, plus turmeric that brings an almost egglike richness, and then spooned over gingery cooked greens or served next to them. Using a duo of sharp-tasting mustard greens and earthy red chard shows how combining two or more kinds of leafy greens can make a dish even better. Serve with Incendiary Herbed Brown Rice (p. 137) or steamed basmati rice.

1 small bunch green or red mustard greens (8 to 10 ounces), center veins and stems removed

1 small bunch red chard (8 to 10 ounces), center veins and stems removed

1 tablespoon cold-pressed sesame oil or canola oil

½ teaspoon black mustard seeds

1 medium onion, finely chopped (1 cup)

2 garlic cloves, finely chopped

1 tablespoon grated ginger

½ teaspoon ground turmeric

¼ teaspoon red pepper flakes, optional

2 tablespoons reduced-fat unsweetened dried coconut

½ teaspoon salt

Lemon Dal (p. 94)

1. Heap the mustard greens and chard together and chop them into roughly 1-inch pieces.

2. In a heavy, large skillet, heat the oil over medium-high heat. Add the mustard seeds and cook, shaking the pan often, until the seeds look gray, 2 to 3 minutes. Add the onion, garlic, ginger, turmeric, and pepper flakes if using. Cook, stirring often, until the onion is golden, about 6 minutes.

3. Add the coconut and half the greens. Cook, stirring, until the leaves are coated with oil and collapsed enough to gradually add the remaining greens. Add ½ cup water and the salt, spread the greens in an even layer, and cook, stirring often, until the greens are crisp-tender, adding water, 2 tablespoons at a time, just to keep the greens simmering gently. When the greens are chewy-tender and almost dry, set them aside.

4. Serve the dal lukewarm, in a bowl beside the greens, spooned over them, or serve the greens and dal together over cooked rice.

LEMON DAL

2/3 cup red lentils

1 medium onion, finely chopped

2 plum tomatoes, seeded and chopped

1 garlic clove, finely chopped

1 teaspoon finely chopped
fresh rosemary

½ teaspoon ground turmeric

Pinch of red pepper flakes

2 cups vegetable broth

1 teaspoon grated lemon zest

Salt and freshly ground pepper

1. In a bowl, rinse the lentils under cold water and drain them, repeating this three or four times, until the water runs almost clear.

2. Place a heavy, large saucepan over medium-high heat. In the dry pot, combine the onion and tomatoes and cook, stirring frequently, until the tomatoes have broken down, 5 minutes. Add the garlic, rosemary, turmeric, and pepper flakes and cook, stirring constantly, for 1 minute.

3. Add the lentils, broth, and 1 cup water. Bring to a boil, reduce the heat to a simmer, cover, and cook until the lentils are tender but still pulpy, 25 minutes. Remove from the heat and mix in the lemon zest and season the dal to taste with salt and pepper. The dal will thicken as it cools.

To store: The dal and greens, combined, keep tightly covered in the refrigerator for 4 days. Reheat in a covered heavy saucepan over medium-high heat, stirring occasionally, until warmed through, about 8 minutes, adding vegetable broth or water, if needed.

NUTRINOTE

Turmeric contains some of nature's most potent anti-inflammatory antioxidants. Eating it is challenging if you did not grow up with its distinctive flavor. Using a little bit at a time and doing it often works best, so I constantly look for subtle ways of adding it. This dal is a good example. I also dissolve a generous pinch in warm water and whisk it into eggs to be scrambled and add one-quarter teaspoon to many soups and stews.

GREEK LENTIL STEW

SERVES 4 |

Greek cooks understand how cinnamon brings elusive, warm, and intriguing flavor to savory dishes. This substantial stew shows how well it melds with tomatoes and chard. Serve with Spicy Chopped Salad (p. 71) or Grilled Romaine Lettuce with Beefsteak Tomatoes and Ranch Dressing (p. 65).

1 medium bunch chard (12 ounces), center veins and stems removed

1 tablespoon extra-virgin olive oil

1 medium red onion, chopped

1 medium orange bell pepper, seeded and chopped

2 garlic cloves, finely chopped

2 teaspoons dried oregano

1 teaspoon ground cinnamon

1 cup green lentils

2½ cups vegetable broth

1 14-ounce can diced tomatoes, preferably fire-roasted

2 teaspoons red wine vinegar

Salt and freshly ground pepper

Crumbled feta cheese, optional, for garnish

1. In a covered, large saucepan, boil 6 cups of water over high heat. Add the chard, pushing it into the water with a wooden spoon. Cover and cook for 4 minutes. Drain the chard in a colander, then run cold water over it while swishing the greens with your hand until they feel cool, 30 seconds. Gather the chard and squeeze it to remove excess water. Chop the chard and pull it apart; there will be about 1½ cups.

2. In a heavy, large saucepan, heat the oil over medium-high heat. Add the onion and pepper, and cook 1 minute, stirring constantly. Cover tightly, reduce the heat to medium-low, and cook for 4 minutes.

3. Increase the heat to medium-high, add the garlic, and cook for 1 minute. Stir in the oregano and cinnamon. Add the lentils, broth, and 1 cup water. When the liquid boils, reduce the heat, cover, and simmer until the lentils are almost tender, about 30 minutes.

4. Add the tomatoes with their liquid. Mix in the chard. Simmer the stew, uncovered, until the lentils and chard are tender, 15 minutes. Let the stew sit, off the heat, for 15 minutes. Stir in the vinegar, and season with salt and pepper.

5. To serve, divide the stew among four bowls. If desired, garnish with crumbled feta cheese.

To store: This dish keeps tightly covered in the refrigerator for 4 days. Reheat it in a covered heavy saucepan over medium-high heat, stirring occasionally, until it is warmed through, about 10 minutes, adding vegetable broth or water, if needed.

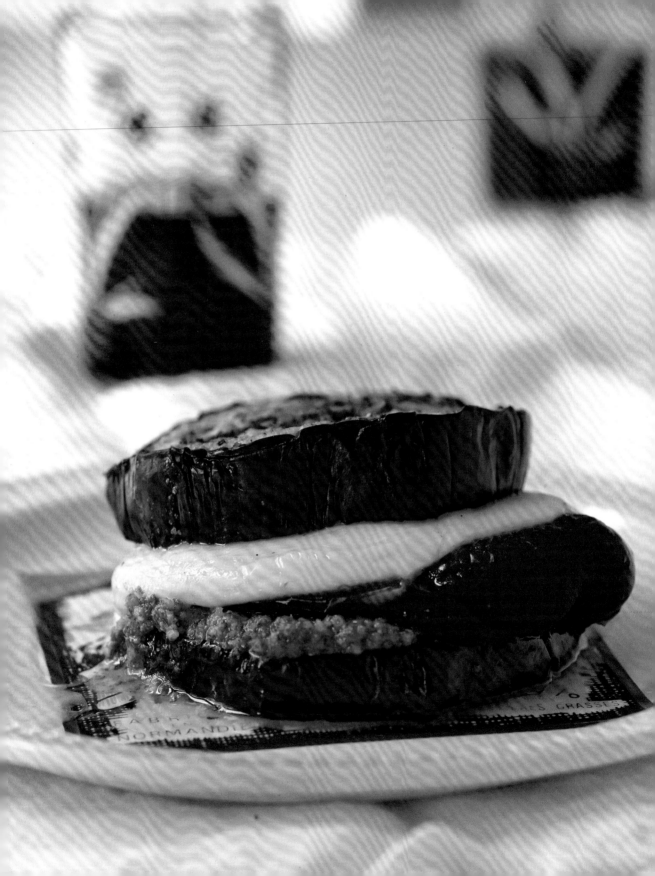

GRILLED EGGPLANT STACKS with RED PEPPER, MOZZARELLA, and ARUGULA PESTO

SERVES 4 |

Instead of making eggplant Parmesan, I prefer the smoky flavor of grilled eggplant layered with mozzarella and roasted peppers in individual stacks. Using a grill pan makes this a dish to prepare anywhere. To keep the slices close in size, so they make neat stacks, look for an eggplant with an elongated shape rather than a bulbous one. Serve with Italian Braised Greens with Roasted Garlic (p. 145) or Caesar Salad with Parmesan Chickpeas (p. 63). For the Arugula Pesto, use the Arugula Pesto, Modified (p. 98), a variation on the recipe from Carrots with Wild Arugula Pesto (p. 173).

2 tablespoons extra-virgin olive oil

2 large red bell peppers, halved lengthwise and seeded

1 medium eggplant, 1¼ to 1½ pounds

4 tablespoons Arugula Pesto, Modified (recipe follows)

4 ½-inch slices fresh mozzarella cheese, or ¾ cup (3 ounces) shredded mozzarella

Salt and freshly ground pepper

1. Preheat the oven to 425°F.

2. Brush a baking sheet with some of the oil. Arrange the peppers on the baking sheet, cut side down, and brush them with oil. Bake for 25 minutes, until their skin is puffy and blistered. Transfer the peppers to a bowl, cover with plastic wrap, and let them steam for 20 minutes. Reduce the oven temperature to 350°F. Set the baking sheet aside. Using your fingers, slip the skins off the peppers.

3. While the peppers steam, set a grill pan over medium-high heat. Cut eight ½-inch slices from the eggplant, slicing them from the part that is most round and even in diameter. Brush the eggplant slices with oil on both sides. Grill the eggplant until the slices are well-marked on both sides, 4 to 6 minutes, using tongs to turn them midway. Continue grilling the eggplant, turning them every 1 to 2 minutes, until the slices look translucent and greenish, 7 to 8 minutes in all. Place the eggplant slices on the baking sheet used for the peppers.

4. Spread 1 tablespoon pesto on four of the eggplant slices. Cover the pesto with a pepper half, trimming it as needed; it can drape over the edge of the eggplant in places but should not hit the baking sheet. Lay a mozzarella slice on top of the

continued on next page

pepper. Sprinkle the cheese with a pinch of salt and several grinds of pepper. Finish each stack with a second eggplant slice. Bake the stacks until the cheese melts, 5 minutes. Serve immediately.

ANOTHER WAY

The unused eggplant is easily turned into the Mediterranean spread baba ganoush. Wrap the eggplant in foil and bake at 400°F until it has collapsed and the flesh is soft, about 45 minutes. Scoop out and mash the warm flesh with tahini, garlic, and lemon juice.

ARUGULA PESTO, MODIFIED

MAKES ⅞ CUP

Arugula Pesto is better with this dish when you substitute roasted garlic and almonds for the shallot and pistachios of the basic recipe in Wild Arugula Pesto (p. 175). Lemon juice adds an edge to the caramelized vegetables and creamy mozzarella. It also keeps this pesto looking bright for several days. Dollop leftover pesto on vegetables, from artichokes or avocado to zucchini, on beans, grilled chicken, or shrimp.

3 packed cups arugula leaves

2 to 3 roasted garlic cloves

⅓ cup slivered almonds

⅓ cup extra-virgin olive oil

1 teaspoon lemon juice

Salt and freshly ground pepper

In a food processor whirl the arugula and garlic cloves until finely chopped. Add the nuts and whirl until the arugula looks moist, about 1 minute. With the motor running, drizzle in the oil, then the lemon juice. Season with salt and pepper. If desired, refrigerate in a tightly covered container for up to 3 days.

POMEGRANATE SHRIMP CURRY

SERVES 4 |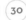

Pomegranate juice is the base of this unusual Indian curry. I discovered it at Vij's restaurant in Vancouver, Canada. A lavish amount of onions cooked to golden sweetness give this dish body while the pomegranate makes it mildly tart. Changing the amounts of ginger and jalapeño pepper used lets you make this dish mild or searing hot. The generous amount of cilantro showered over this curry is an essential part of its flavor. Serve with basmati rice and a dark, leafy green, perhaps the mustard greens from Indian Greens with Lemon Dal (p. 93).

2 tablespoons coconut oil

½ teaspoon cumin seeds

1½ cups finely chopped red onions

¼ teaspoon ground turmeric

¼ teaspoon freshly ground pepper

1 small jalapeño pepper, finely chopped

2 teaspoons grated ginger

1 teaspoon salt

½ cup pomegranate juice

¾ pound medium (41- to 50-count) shrimp, shelled and deveined

½ cup chopped cilantro

1. In a medium skillet, heat the oil over medium-high heat. Add the cumin seeds and fry until they turn golden brown, 45 seconds, watching carefully. Add the onions and cook, stirring often, until they are golden and just starting to brown, 8 minutes.

2. Mix in the turmeric and black pepper. Add the jalapeño, ginger, and salt and cook, stirring, for 1 minute. Pour in the pomegranate juice. When the juice boils, add the shrimp, reduce the heat, and simmer until the shrimp look pink outside and are white in the center, 4 minutes. Remove from the heat and mix in the cilantro, reserving 2 tablespoons to sprinkle on top as a garnish.

COOK'S TIP

Using frozen shrimp is fine in this light curry. Look for brands containing only salt, without sulfites or other additives. Small (51- to 60-count) white shrimp are actually nice here as well as being less expensive.

RED CHILI TOFU with BABY BOK CHOY

SERVES 4 | **GF** **30**

These tofu cutlets will ignite your hot spot. Their heat comes from Chinese chili paste (preferably Lum Chi brand, available at Asian markets). Serving the tofu on a bed of stir-fried baby bok choy adds succulence and color. Start your meal with cool Spinach Gazpacho with Walnuts (p. 57) or Mulligatawny Soup with Mustard Greens (p. 50).

1 (14- to 19-ounce) package firm tofu

2 tablespoons chili paste with garlic

1 tablespoon honey, preferably mesquite

2 teaspoons reduced-sodium soy sauce

2 tablespoons fresh lime juice

½ teaspoon sugar

½ teaspoon salt

⅓ cup fat-free reduced-sodium chicken broth

1 tablespoon peanut oil

½ inch ginger, thinly sliced

12 small heads baby bok choy, about 1¼ pounds, halved lengthwise, rinsed, and dried

2 tablespoons coarsely chopped cilantro, for garnish

1. Cut the tofu into 8 slices. Press the tofu for 10 minutes (see p. 101).

2. For the tofu marinade, in an 11 x 7-inch baking dish or a platter large enough to hold the tofu in one layer, combine the chili paste, honey, soy sauce, and lime juice. One at a time, add the tofu slices, turning to coat them on all sides with the marinade before adding the next slice. Set the tofu aside to marinate while making the bok choy.

3. In a small bowl, combine the sugar, salt, and broth, whisking until the sugar dissolves. In a heavy, large skillet, heat the oil over high heat. Add the ginger and stir-fry until it is fragrant, 30 seconds. Heap the bok choy into the pan; it will mound very high. Using tongs, lift some of the bok choy from the bottom of the heap, turn it over, and set it back on top of the heap. Keep doing this until all the bok choy has collapsed, looks shiny, and is bright green, about 3 minutes. Pour in the broth mixture and stir-fry until the bok choy is tender-crisp, 3 to 4 minutes. Using tongs, transfer the bok choy to a serving platter. Pour off the liquid in the pan and wipe the pan out.

4. Return the pan to medium-high heat. Arrange the marinated tofu in the dry pan in one layer and cook until seared and lightly colored on the bottom, 2 minutes. Turn the tofu, using tongs, and cook until lightly colored on the second side, 1 to 2 minutes. Arrange the tofu on top of the bok choy. Sprinkle on the cilantro, and serve.

To store: Leftover tofu keeps tightly covered in the refrigerator for 3 days. So does extra stir-fried bok choy, which should be stored separately. Serve leftovers at room temperature, which is the Asian way.

NUTRINOTE

The heat in chile peppers comes from capsaicin. Along with its other benefits, it is antibacterial.

TO PRESS TOFU

Line a baking sheet with three layers of paper towels. Arrange sliced tofu on the baking sheet almost touching one another. Cover with two layers of paper towels, then place another baking sheet on top of the tofu. Weight the tofu by setting four large cans (tomatoes or beans work well) on top of the baking sheet. Or use two large cans, then place a cast-iron skillet on top of them. If not using it immediately, store the pressed tofu, covered with water, in the refrigerator for 2 to 3 days. Save the paper towels, drying them out and reusing them.

TOFU PICCATA with SAUTÉED SPINACH

SERVES 4 | 30

The nutty taste of tofu that some people find bland is a virtue here, letting you fully taste the piquant lemon sauce in this dish. Garlic-sharpened spinach is its ideal accompaniment. Serve with Quinoa Pilaf with Carrots and Kale Stems (p. 132), or steamed basmati rice.

One 14-ounce package extra-firm tofu

1 tablespoon capers, preferably salt-preserved

3 tablespoons extra-virgin olive oil, divided

3 roasted garlic cloves

1 bunch flat-leaf spinach

⅓ cup fresh lemon juice

⅓ cup dry white wine, such as Sauvignon Blanc

⅓ cup fat-free reduced-sodium chicken broth

¼ cup unbleached all-purpose flour

¼ cup plain dry bread crumbs

Salt and freshly ground pepper

4 thin lemon slices, optional, for garnish

1. Cut the tofu into 8 slices. Press the tofu for 10 minutes (see p. 101).

2. Meanwhile, in a small bowl, soak the capers in cold water for 20 minutes. Stem the spinach, rinse well in cold water, and dry the leaves.

3. For the spinach, in a large skillet, heat 1 tablespoon of the oil over medium-high heat. Mash the garlic in the oil. Add the spinach and stir until it collapses, 2 minutes. Cook until the spinach is tender, 3 to 4 minutes, stirring constantly. Divide the spinach among four plates. Wipe out the pan.

4. Drain the capers. In a measuring cup, combine the lemon juice, wine, and broth. For the tofu, in a wide, shallow dish, combine the flour and breadcrumbs, ½ teaspoon salt, and 6 grinds of pepper. One at a time, dredge the tofu slices in the flour mixture, coating them on both sides, and place them in the pan in one layer. When the tofu is browned in places on the bottom, 3 minutes, turn and brown it lightly on the other side, 3 minutes. Using a wide spatula, arrange 2 tofu slices against the spinach on each plate.

5. Pour the lemon and wine mixture into the pan, scraping the bottom of the pan with a wooden spoon as the liquid boils to gather up any browned bits. Boil until the liquid is reduced to ½ cup, about 4 minutes. Add the capers. Spoon one-fourth of the lemon sauce over the tofu and spinach. Garnish each plate with a lemon slice, if using, and serve.

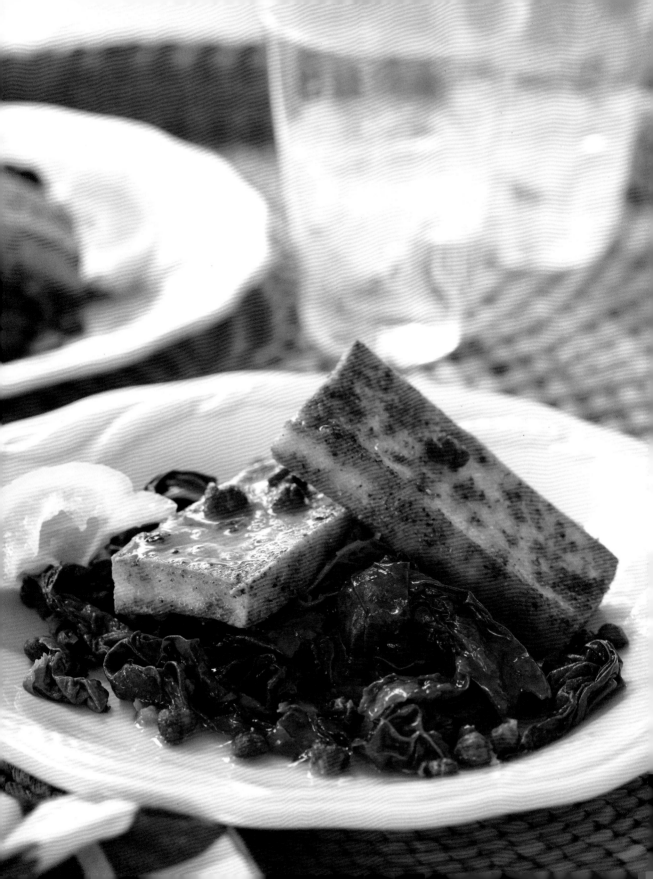

COD with ROASTED EGGPLANT RATATOUILLE

SERVES 4 |

Oven-roasted ratatouille is ideal to serve with cod and other meaty white fish. Using a pan that can go from stovetop to oven, you cook the ratatouille and the fish all in one pot. Placing the fish on top of the vegetables keeps it moist while the ratatouille still keeps its individual flavor. This dish is easy to make when cooking for one and also a good choice to share with company. Serve it with braised chard or Chard with Browned Onions (p. 156). Both go well with the fish while providing stems to use in the ratatouille. Make the ratatouille without the cod, and mix in French green lentils for a meatless main dish.

3 tablespoons plus 1 teaspoon extra-virgin olive oil

1 cup chopped shallots

4 cups Asian eggplant, in ½-inch cubes

1 cup thinly sliced white chard stems

1 medium red bell pepper, seeded and chopped (about 1 cup)

Salt and freshly ground pepper

4 4- to 6-ounce pieces fresh cod fillets

1. Preheat the oven to 400°F.

2. In a large skillet that can go into the oven, heat the 3 tablespoons of oil. When the oil is hot, add the shallots and cook, stirring occasionally, until they are translucent, 4 minutes. Add the eggplant, chard stems, and red pepper, and cook, stirring occasionally, until the eggplant is soft, 5 minutes. Season with salt and pepper.

3. Brush the pieces of cod with the 1 teaspoon of oil and season with salt and pepper. Lay the fish on top of the eggplant mixture, placing the pieces a few inches apart. Transfer the skillet to the oven.

4. Roast until the cod flakes easily and is opaque white in the center at the thickest part, 12 to 15 minutes, depending on the thickness of the fish.

5. To serve, use a wide spatula to transfer one-fourth of the ratatouille and a piece of the cod to each of four plates.

To store: The ratatouille keeps covered in the refrigerator for 4 days. Serve it at room temperature, adjusting the seasoning with salt and pepper.

SALMON STEAMED in a CABBAGE LEAF with CORN BUTTER

SERVES 4 |

A head of Savoy cabbage is one of nature's loveliest creations. Throwing away its outer leaves made me feel guilty until I found a way to discard only the very first, most leathery layer and use the leaves just under it as a wrap for cooking salmon. The result is exquisitely soft and moist. This French-American version of *beurre blanc,* made with lemon juice and sweet corn, complements the salmon beautifully. If white corn is available, fresh or frozen, using it is ideal.

4 Savoy cabbage outer leaves, 7 to 8 inches from base to tip

4 6-ounce salmon fillets, skinned

Salt and freshly ground pepper

1 ear corn, kernels removed, or ½ cup frozen corn, preferably white

2 tablespoons very finely chopped shallots

1 tablespoon fresh lemon juice

3 tablespoons unsalted butter, finely chopped, and chilled

1. In a large saucepan of hot water, simmer the cabbage leaves gently until they are flexible and almost tender but still slightly chewy, 6 to 10 minutes. Using tongs, lift, shake, and transfer the leaves, one at a time, to a work surface and pat them dry. Pour off the cabbage water, leaving 1½ inches in the pot, and set aside.

2. Place a cabbage leaf facedown, so the prominent rib faces you. Holding a sharp small knife horizontally, shave the rib almost flat, so you can bend the bottom of the leaf up. Place a piece of salmon crosswise in the center of the leaf, and season it with a pinch of salt and 3 grinds of pepper. Fold the cabbage leaf like a burrito to envelop the salmon, starting with the bottom. When folded down, the top of the leaf should reach over the salmon and down the side. Repeat to wrap the other pieces.

3. Place a steamer insert in the saucepan with the cabbage water, cover, and bring the water to a boil. Add the salmon packets, cover, and steam until an instant-read thermometer inserted into the center of the thickest part registers 125°F, 10 to 12 minutes, depending on the thickness of the fish. Using tongs, transfer the fish to four dinner plates.

4. While the salmon steams, for the sauce, in a small saucepan, combine the corn with ½ cup water. Cook over medium-high heat, uncovered, until the corn is tender and just moist, 8 to 10 minutes. Add the shallots, lemon juice,

continued on page 107

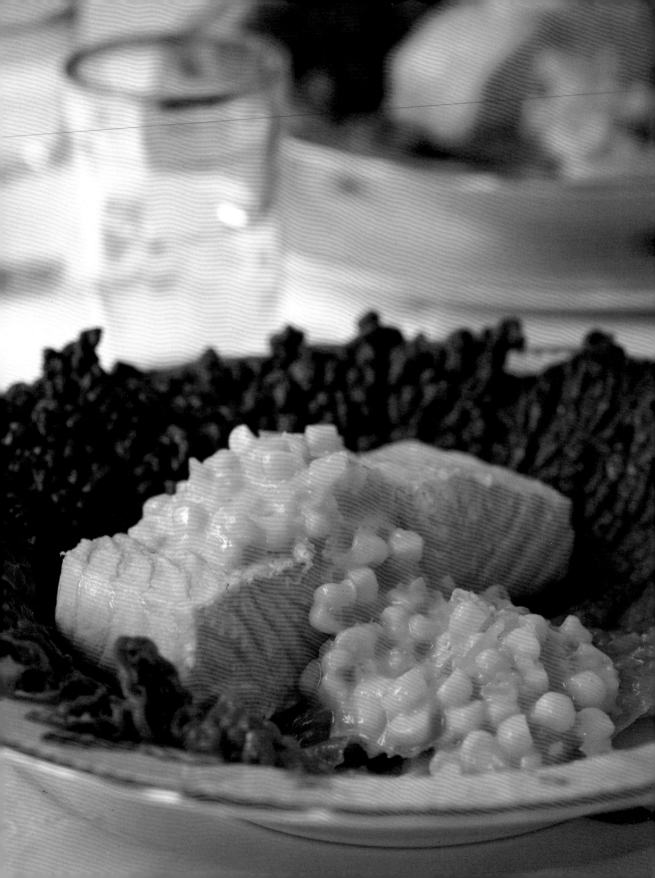

and 1 teaspoon water, and simmer until most of the liquid has evaporated, 2 minutes. Reduce the heat to low. While whisking, add the chilled butter, a few pieces at a time, waiting until it melts and the sauce looks creamy before adding more butter. Remove from the heat and season the corn butter to taste with salt and pepper. There will be about ¾ cup corn butter.

5. To serve, spoon one-fourth of the corn butter alongside the salmon.

COOK'S TIPS

Using a Savoy cabbage that has all its leaves, removing 3 or 4 leaves gets you to the right layer, where the leaves are firm but not leathery.
Cook and and trim the cabbage leaves up to a day ahead then refrigerate them wrapped in plastic, and this dish will be ready to serve in 30 minutes.

After cutting the corn kernels off the cob, scrape the cob with the back of the knife and add the creamy corn milk to the kernels.

I like the responsibly farmed salmon from Scotland. If you use wild coho or sockeye, it cooks faster so reduce the cooking time. It also gives a drier result.

PAN-SEARED CHICKEN CUTLETS with ARUGULA, ORANGE, and FENNEL

SERVES 4 |

Warm chicken served over a Sicilian salad of greens and citrus demonstrates how a simple dish can outshine more elaborate ones. Pounding the chicken evenly thin is important. So is using enough oil to prevent the very lean chicken from drying out.

2 navel oranges

1 medium fennel bulb

2 packed cups baby or wild arugula leaves

2 small red onions, sliced into thin rounds

Salt and freshly ground pepper

4 tablespoons extra-virgin olive oil, divided

4 (4- to 6-ounce) skinless and boneless chicken cutlets

1. Peel the oranges, using a sharp knife to cut away the rind and white pith. Slice each orange into 8 rounds, setting aside the top and bottom slices. Cut off and discard the fennel stalks and feathery tops. Halve the bulb vertically. Cut off a slice from the bottom and remove any tough outer layers. Cut the fennel crosswise into thin slices and place the slices in a mixing bowl.

2. Make a bed of the arugula on four dinner plates. Arrange one-fourth of the fennel slices on one side of the plate. Top with 3 orange slices and some red onion, separated into rings.

3. For the dressing, squeeze the reserved orange slices over a small bowl. Whisk in ½ teaspoon salt, several grinds of pepper, and 2 tablespoons of the olive oil.

4. Place each chicken cutlet, one at a time, between two sheets of wax paper and pound it with the flat side of a meat mallet until it is evenly ¼-inch thick; if the cutlets are very thick or uneven, turning them over 3 or 4 times will help. Brush the cutlets with olive oil, using 1 tablespoon, and season them on each side with a pinch of salt and a grind of pepper.

5. In a large skillet, heat 1 tablespoon of the oil over medium-high heat. Add the chicken cutlets and cook until they are golden brown, 5 minutes. Turn and lightly brown the chicken on the second side. You may have to do this in two batches.

6. To serve, place a cooked chicken cutlet on top of the arugula, letting it also cover part of the fennel and oranges. Spoon the dressing over the chicken, and serve.

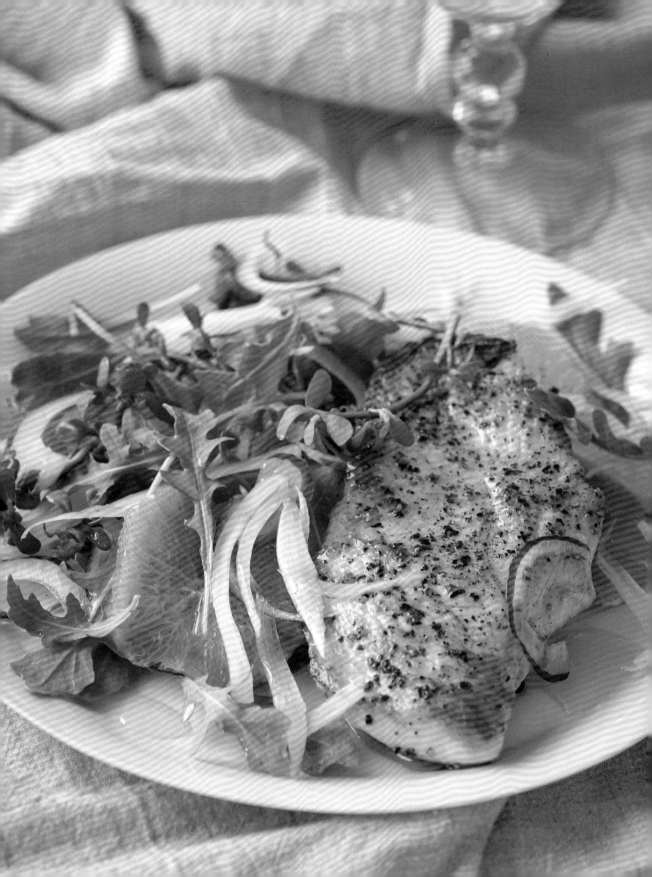

TURKEY HASH with SWEET POTATOES and GREENS

SERVES 4 | GF

Hash was created to use up leftovers but this colorful one is so good that it's worth making from scratch. Gentle on the budget, it provides health benefits from almost every food group—protein, carbs, and a little healthy fat, nutrient-dense green and orange vegetables, plus alliums, herbs, and spices. Serve an Oatmeal Everything Cookie (p. 208) and Parsley-Ginger Lemonade (p. 214) for dessert.

1 medium bunch (12 ounces) red chard, Tuscan kale, or a combination of dark greens, center vein and stems removed

3 cups coarsely shredded orange-fleshed sweet potatoes, such as Jewel, Garnet, or Beauregard

2 tablespoons plus 1 teaspoon canola oil

1 medium onion, chopped (1 cup)

1 large garlic clove

12 ounces 93% lean ground turkey

1 teaspoon dried thyme

½ teaspoon smoked paprika

Cayenne pepper

Salt and freshly ground pepper

⅓ cup chopped scallions, green part only

1. In a covered, large saucepan, boil 6 cups of water over high heat. Add the chard, pushing it into the water with a wooden spoon. Cook, covered, for 4 minutes; 6 minutes if using kale. Drain the chard in a colander, then run cold water over it while swishing the leaves with your hand until they feel cool, 30 seconds. Gather the chard and squeeze it to remove excess water; if necessary do this in several handfuls. Chop the chard and pull it apart; there will be about 1½ cups chopped chard or 2 cups kale.

2. In a mixing bowl, toss the shredded potatoes with 4 teaspoons of the oil until they are evenly coated.

3. In a large skillet, heat the remaining tablespoon of oil over medium-high heat. Add the onion and cook, stirring occasionally, until it is translucent, 4 minutes. Add the garlic and cook for 1 minute. Add the ground turkey and cook, using a wooden spoon to break it up, until it loses its pink color, 8 minutes. Mix in the potatoes, chopped greens, and thyme, and cook, stirring occasionally, until the potatoes and greens are almost tender, 12 minutes. Add the paprika and a pinch of cayenne pepper, and cook until the potatoes are soft, 3 minutes. Season with salt and pepper.

4. To serve, divide the hash among four dinner plates and garnish with the scallions.

To store: This dish will keep for 3 days tightly covered in the refrigerator. It is perfect reheated as leftovers sealed in foil and baked at 350°F for 20 minutes for one serving, 30 minutes for two servings.

COOK'S TIP

Coating shredded potatoes with oil helps to keep them from sticking to the pan and making a mess. It works with any kind of potato.

PICK THE PROPER SWEET POTATO

Sweet potatoes can have orange, bright yellow, creamy white, or purple flesh. (The lighter-fleshed kinds that are sometimes called yams are actually sweet potatoes, too.) Orange-fleshed Garnet or Jewel yams or Beauregard sweet potatoes are the ones to use in recipes here.

TURKEY SAUSAGE and PEPPERS with SPIGARIELLO

SERVES 4 |

To fit more dark, leafy greens into the day I add them to dishes where you do not usually find them—but only when they work with the rest of the dish. Spigariello, the Italian leaf broccoli, is a good example, melding right in with the sausages and peppers. Broccoli leaves or Tuscan kale are equally good when spigariello is not available. The green frying peppers called Cubanelle and red ones called field peppers are ideal in this dish. Serve with Quinoa Pilaf with Carrots and Kale Stems (p. 132).

1 bunch spigariello, broccoli leaf, or Tuscan kale (8 to 10 ounces), center veins and stems removed

3 tablespoons extra-virgin olive oil

4 links sweet or hot Italian turkey sausage

3 garlic cloves, smashed and peeled

1 large red onion, halved and cut into 16 wedges

3 large green Cubanelle peppers, seeded and cut into 3/4-inch strips

2 large red bell peppers, seeded and cut into 3/4-inch strips

1 teaspoon salt

Freshly ground black pepper

1. Cut the spigariello leaves crosswise into thin strips. In a covered, large saucepan, boil 4 cups of water over high heat. Add the spigariello, pushing it into the water with a wooden spoon. Cook, covered, for 4 minutes. Drain the spigariello in a colander, then run cold water over it while swishing the greens with your hand until they feel cool, 30 seconds. Gather the greens and squeeze them to remove excess water. Pull the compressed greens apart; there will be about 1¼ cups. See Note if using Tuscan kale.

2. In a large skillet, heat 1 tablespoon of the oil over medium-high heat. Add the sausage and brown it on all sides, 10 to 12 minutes, using tongs to turn the sausage every 2 minutes. Set the sausage aside. Wipe out the pan.

3. Return the pan to medium-high heat. Add the remaining 2 tablespoons of oil. Add the garlic and cook until lightly browned on all sides, about 3 minutes. Discard the garlic.

4. Add the onion and cook, stirring occasionally, until it is limp, 3 minutes. Add the peppers, stirring to coat them with oil. Cook for 5 minutes, stirring occasionally. Add 1 cup water, and as it boils, use a wooden spatula to scrape and gather up the browned bits from the bottom of the pan. Add the spigariello and sausage, including any juices from the plate. Cook, stirring and scraping the bottom of the pan occasionally, until the spigariello is tender and the sausage is cooked through, about 20 minutes. Season with salt and pepper.

To store: This dish will keep tightly covered in the refrigerator for 3 days. Reheat it in a foil-covered baking dish, adding a splash of water, at 350°F for 20 to 30 minutes, depending on the number of servings.

USING TUSCAN KALE

Stem and remove the center veins from a small bunch of Tuscan kale (8 to 10 ounces). Cut the leaves crosswise into ¾-inch strips.

In a large covered saucepan, boil 6 cups of water over high heat. Add the kale, pushing it into the water with a wooden spoon. Cook, covered, for 6 minutes. Drain the kale in a colander, then run cold water over it while swishing it with your hand until it feels cool, 30 seconds. Gather the kale and squeeze it to remove excess water. Pull the compressed kale apart; there will be about 1 cup.

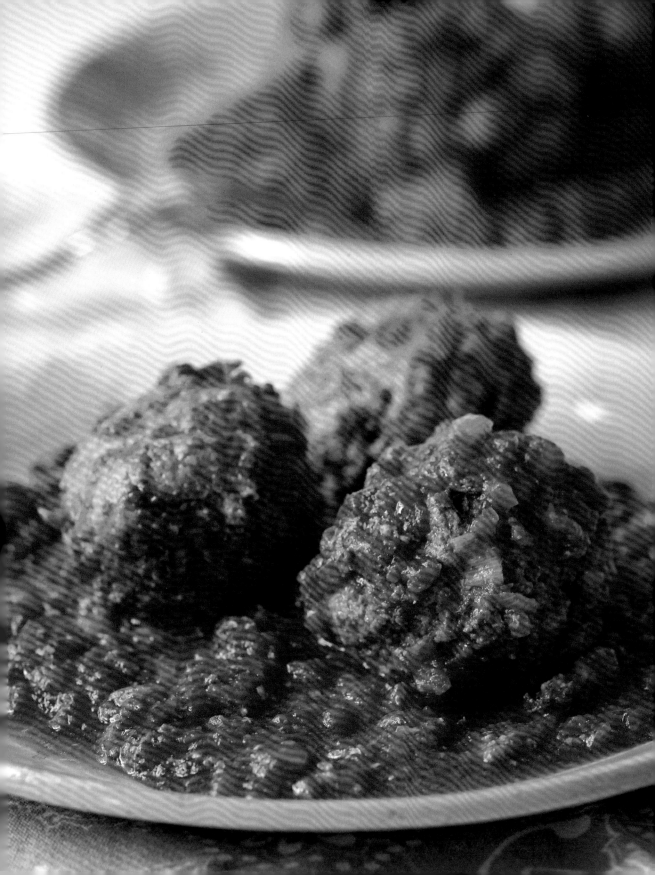

MEATBALLS with RED PEPPER TOMATO SAUCE

SERVES 4

When I was a teenager, a friend's Italian *nonna* taught me how to make tender, juicy meatballs. I still hear her admonishing *delicatamente* as she shaped loosely knit, slightly irregular balls and softly dropped them into the simmering red sauce she called gravy. Mixing broccoli rabe into the meat helps keep it moist. I also amp up the sauce by including a roasted red pepper. Serve these meatballs in a bowl, bathed in sauce, or on top of spaghetti, rigatoni, or cooked rice, starting the meal with Caesar Salad with Parmesan Chickpeas (p. 63).

1 tablespoon extra-virgin olive oil

1 medium onion, chopped

3 roasted garlic cloves

1 28-ounce can plum tomatoes

1 large roasted red pepper, chopped (about ½ cup)

1 teaspoon salt

Pinch of sugar, optional

Freshly ground pepper

½ cup tomato sauce

. . . . . .

4 packed cups broccoli rabe leaves

2 teaspoons extra-virgin olive oil

1 small onion, finely chopped (½ cup)

1 small garlic clove, finely chopped

1 pound 90 to 93% lean ground beef

⅓ cup dry breadcrumbs

3 tablespoons grated pecorino cheese

½ teaspoon salt

Freshly ground pepper

1 large egg, plus 1 egg white

1. For the sauce, in a large saucepan, heat the oil over medium-high heat. Add the onion and cook until it is translucent, 4 minutes, stirring occasionally. Stir in the garlic and cook for 1 minute. Add the tomatoes, one at a time, holding them over the pot in your fist and squeezing to squish them and letting the juices fall into the pot. Add the liquid from the can, the roasted red pepper, salt, sugar, if using, and three or four grinds pepper, as well as the tomato sauce. Simmer the sauce for 20 minutes, reducing the heat as needed.

2. In a covered, large saucepan, boil 6 cups of water over high heat. Add the broccoli rabe leaves, pushing them into the water with a wooden spoon. Cook, covered, for 5 minutes. Drain the broccoli rabe in a colander, then run cold water over it while swishing the leaves with your hand until they feel cool, 30 seconds. Gather the leaves and squeeze them to remove excess water. Chop the broccoli rabe and pull it apart; there will be about 1 cup.

3. While the sauce simmers, in a small skillet, heat the oil. Add the onion and garlic, and cook, stirring often, until the onion is translucent, 4 minutes. Using a large spoon, transfer them to a medium mixing bowl. Add the meat, breadcrumbs, cheese, salt, and pepper. Slide the egg and egg white down the side of the bowl, beat with a fork, then mix to combine the

continued on next page

meatball mixture. Mix in the broccoli rabe. Divide the meat into 12 portions and form into 12 loosely knit meatballs.

4. Remove from the heat and use an immersion blender to blend the sauce to a pulpy puree. Add the meatballs to the pot of sauce, arranging them in one layer. Return the pot to the heat and simmer gently until the meatballs are no longer pink in the center, 20 minutes.

5. Serve the meatballs alone, over spaghetti, or on top of brown rice, accompanied by Italian Braised Greens with Roasted Garlic (p. 145).

To store: The meatballs and sauce keep, stored separately and tightly covered in the refrigerator, for up to 3 days. To reheat, arrange the meatballs in one layer in a baking dish, add the sauce, cover with foil, and bake at 350°F until the meatballs are hot in the center, 30 to 40 minutes. Bringing the meatballs and sauce to room temperature before reheating them is best.

ANOTHER WAY

For the broccoli rabe to melt into the meatballs, use only the leaves. Using just the leaves lets the broccoli rabe melt into the meatballs. For the florets and stems, cook them as in Italian Braised Greens with Roasted Garlic (p. 145). Serve them along with the meatballs or save them to serve with extra sauce from the meatballs on top of farro spaghetti or whole-wheat pasta.

KALE-SMOTHERED PORK CHOPS
with CARROT and APPLE

SERVES 4 | GF

This one-pot, easy dish provides moist chops and generous servings of tender kale braised with sweet apple and colorful carrot. When cooking for two, leftovers are great to pack up for lunches. Today's pork is so lean that the bit of fat on bone-in chops is welcome. Usually, chops are smothered during cooking. Here, braising them on top of the kale, then serving them smothered under a heap of it makes for juicier chops.

4 bone-in center-cut loin pork chops, ¾-inch thick

Salt

2 tablespoons extra-virgin olive oil

1 medium onion, halved and thinly sliced

1 medium carrot, cut into ½-inch slices

1 medium bunch green curly kale (10 to 12 ounces), stemmed and coarsely chopped

1 Gala apple, peeled, quartered, and sliced crosswise

1½ teaspoons dried thyme

½ teaspoon caraway seeds

½ cup fat-free, reduced-sodium chicken broth

Freshly ground pepper

1. Season the chops lightly with salt. In a deep skillet over medium-high heat, heat 1 tablespoon of the oil. Brown the pork chops on both sides, about 4 minutes per side. Transfer the chops to a plate.

2. Add the remaining 1 tablespoon oil to the pan. Add the onion and carrot and cook until the onion is limp, 4 minutes, stirring occasionally. Mix in the kale and apple, pushing the kale with a wooden spoon until it collapses. When the kale is moist, scrape the browned bits from the bottom of the pan.

3. Mix in the thyme and caraway seeds, then add the broth. Arrange the chops on top of the kale. Cover and simmer until the chops are white in the center, 30 minutes.

4. To serve, place each chop on a plate. Season the kale with salt and pepper and mound it on top of the chops.

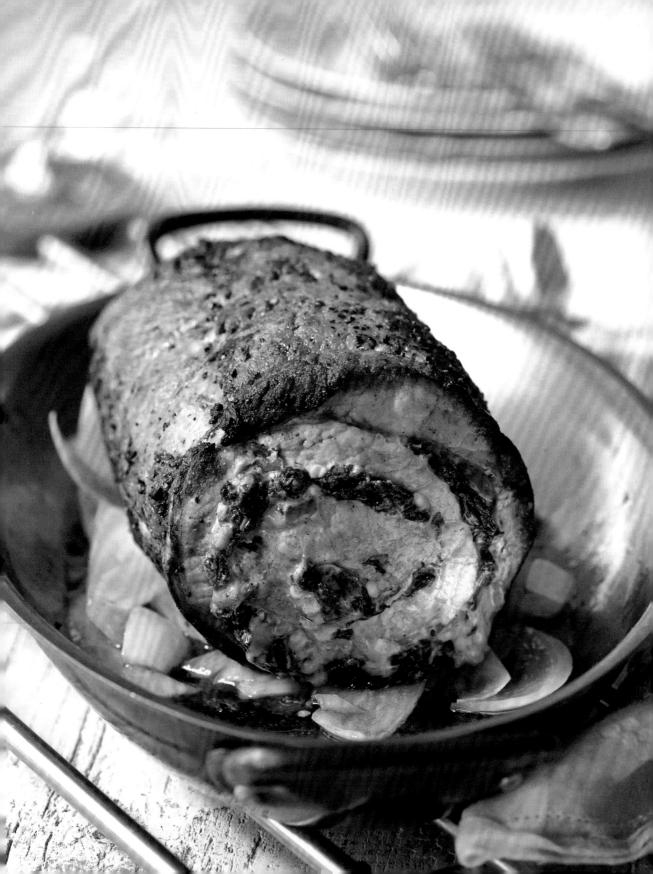

"PORCHETTA" ROAST PORK LOIN STUFFED with BROCCOLI RABE

SERVES 6 | (GF)

This is one of my all-time favorite recipes. The idea for it evolved as I thought about the rosemary, sage, and fennel seasoning rubbed over porchetta, the whole pig that Italians roast in its skin. Here I use this seasoning blend on a pork loin that I flatten, stuff, and roll up like a flank steak. Share it with friends or, since leftovers keep well, enjoy it all for yourself, one slice at a time. On a day when you decide to stay inside and invest yourself in cooking something special, the aroma as this roast cooks will have every mouth in the house watering in anticipation. With the florets not used in this dish, make Tortelloni with Broccoli Rabe Florets (p. 131).

2 pounds boneless center-cut pork loin

SEASONING PASTE

1 teaspoon coriander seed

1 teaspoon fennel seed

1 tablespoon finely chopped fresh rosemary

1 tablespoon finely chopped fresh sage

2 teaspoons kosher salt

2 tablespoons extra-virgin olive oil

1 teaspoon grated lemon zest

FILLING

½ bunch broccoli rabe (about ¾ pound), florets and coarse stems removed

2 tablespoons extra-virgin olive oil

½ cup finely chopped red onion

1 garlic clove, finely chopped

⅓ cup finely chopped peeled Fuji apple

Salt and freshly ground pepper

1. Place the pork on a work surface with the thin layer of fat on the top and a cut end toward you. Holding a sharp knife with the blade tilted down at a 45-degree angle, make a 1-inch-deep cut about one-third of the way up from the bottom along the long, more tapered side of the loin. Turn the knife blade parallel to the cutting board and keep making 1-inch cuts lengthwise while using your other hand to lift the meat so you can keep making cuts. This lets you open the loin like a jelly roll until it becomes a flat sheet more or less even in thickness. Do not worry about small ridges or ragged cuts—trust me that they will disappear when the meat is stuffed and rolled. If there is an extra bulge of meat at one of the ends, flatten it out by making some shorter slits.

2. For the seasoning paste, in a mini food processor, pulse the coriander and fennel seeds to chop them finely. Add the rosemary, sage, and salt and whirl for 5 seconds. With the motor running, add the oil. Mix in the lemon zest. Rub the meat all over with the seasoning paste. Roll it up along the long side, wrap the roast in plastic wrap, and marinate it in the refrigerator for 4 to 24 hours. An hour before stuffing and roasting the pork, bring it to room temperature.

continued on next page

1 large yellow onion, cut into ½-inch wedges

¼ cup hard apple cider

¾ cup sweet apple cider

1½ teaspoons finely chopped fresh sage

4 shallots, thinly sliced (½ cup)

3. Preheat the oven to 350°F.

4. For the filling, chop the broccoli rabe leaves and stems. In a covered, large saucepan, boil 8 cups of water. Add the rabe and cook, uncovered, until tender, 4 minutes. Drain the broccoli rabe in a colander, then run cold water over it while swishing with your hand until it feels cool, 30 seconds. Gather the broccoli rabe and gently squeeze it to remove excess water. Finely chop the compressed greens, then pull them apart and place the broccoli rabe in a mixing bowl. There will be about ¾ cup.

5. In a medium skillet, heat 4 teaspoons of the oil. Add the red onion and cook, stirring frequently, until it is translucent, 4 minutes. Mix in the garlic, broccoli rabe, and apple, and cook, stirring occasionally, until the onion is soft, 3 minutes. Season with salt and pepper. After making the filling, do not clean the pan.

6. To stuff the roast, first cut five 15-inch lengths of kitchen twine. Unroll the meat and wipe off the seasoning paste. Spread the filling to cover the meat, leaving 1 inch on all sides. Lifting the bottom edge, roll up the roast, pressing the filling to keep it in place as you work. Tie the roast, first 1 inch in from each end, then at 1-inch intervals. Pack any extra filling into the ends.

7. Distribute the yellow onion wedges over the bottom of a roasting pan slightly larger than the roast. Pour in ½ cup water. Heat the remaining 2 teaspoons of oil in the skillet already used to make the filling. Brown the tied roast on all sides, using tongs to turn it every 2 minutes, 8 to 10 minutes in all. Place the roast in the prepared roasting pan and bake until the internal temperature at the center reaches 140°F, about 40 minutes. Remove the roast from the oven, transfer it to a platter, cover loosely with foil, and let it sit for 15 minutes. During this time, the internal temperature of the pork will rise to 145°F.

8. For the sauce, return the skillet used for browning the roast to medium-high heat. Pour in the hard cider and as it boils scrape the pan with a wooden spoon to gather up the browned bits. When the hard cider is reduced to 2 tablespoons, 2 minutes, add the sweet cider, any juices accumulated around the resting roast, plus the sage and shallots. Simmer vigorously until the sauce is reduced to ½ cup, 4 minutes.

9. To serve, cut the roast into twelve ½-inch slices and arrange them on a serving platter. Spoon the cider sauce over the meat.

To store: Leftovers are so good that you will be happy serving this roast when it is freshly made and having the rest as leftovers. It will keep covered in the refrigerator for 4 days.

GOOD TECHNIQUE

Using the same skillet to make the filling, brown the roast, and finally to make the sauce produces concentrated layers of flavor that meld together, giving this dish its aromatic, savory, and sweet beauty.

ANOTHER WAY

The onion from the roasting pan is far too good to discard. Use it, and the pan juices, to flavor a soup, stew, or a pot of lentils. Chop the slightly firm onion, then store it along with the liquid in a covered container in the refrigerator for up to 4 days.

GINGER BEEF with BOK CHOY

SERVES 4

Including bok choy in this Chinese favorite brings it closer to the way Asians eat, using a generous amount of vegetables in dishes made with meat. You want the robust flavor and firm crispness of mature bok choy, not milder tasting, more tender baby or Shanghai bok choy.

Remember that cutting the ingredients into similar size pieces so they cook evenly is key for a successful stir-fry.

8 ounces flank steak

2 tablespoons plus 1 teaspoon reduced-sodium soy sauce

1 tablespoon plus 2 teaspoons rice wine or dry sherry

1/4 teaspoon salt

3/4 pound bok choy

2 to 3 inches fresh ginger

2 1/2 teaspoons cornstarch, divided

1/2 teaspoon sugar

2 tablespoons peanut oil, divided

2 garlic cloves, sliced

1. Cut the beef with the grain into 2-inch-wide strips. Cut the strips across the grain into 1/4-inch slices. In a medium bowl, combine the meat with 1 teaspoon of the soy sauce, 2 teaspoons of the rice wine, and the salt. Set the meat aside to marinate for 15 minutes.

2. Meanwhile, separate the bok choy into stalks. Cut the white part of the bok choy diagonally into 1/2-inch slices. Save the dark, leafy top part to use in juice or a vegetable stir-fry. Slice the ginger into thin rounds. Two or three slices at a time, stack the rounds, then cut them crosswise to make thin shreds.

3. For the sauce, in a small bowl, combine 2 tablespoons soy sauce, 1 tablespoon rice wine, 1 teaspoon cornstarch, and the sugar. Sprinkle the remaining 1 1/2 teaspoons cornstarch over the meat, mixing to coat it.

4. Heat a wok over high heat until water flecked into it instantly beads and bounces. Swirl in 1 tablespoon of the oil. Add the beef, spreading it in one layer. Cook for 20 seconds, until the meat starts to brown. Using a metal spatula, stir-fry the meat until it is no longer red, about 2 minutes. Transfer the beef to a plate.

5. Swirl the remaining 1 tablespoon of oil into the wok. Add the garlic and stir-fry for 30 seconds. Add the bok choy and stir-fry 1 to 2 minutes, until the green bits of the bok choy are bright, shiny green. Add the beef. Restir the seasoning sauce, add it to the wok, and stir-fry until the sauce thickens,

about 30 seconds. Serve immediately, accompanied by cooked rice, if you wish.

To store: This dish will keep tightly covered in the refrigerator for 2 days. Asians serve stir-fry leftovers at room temperature rather than overcooking them as they reheat. I agree, letting the leftovers from this dish sit out for 20 minutes and then serving them over freshly cooked hot rice.

GOOD TECHNIQUE

To make slicing easier, place the beef in the freezer until almost firm, about 1 hour. Use a sharp knife to cut the meat.

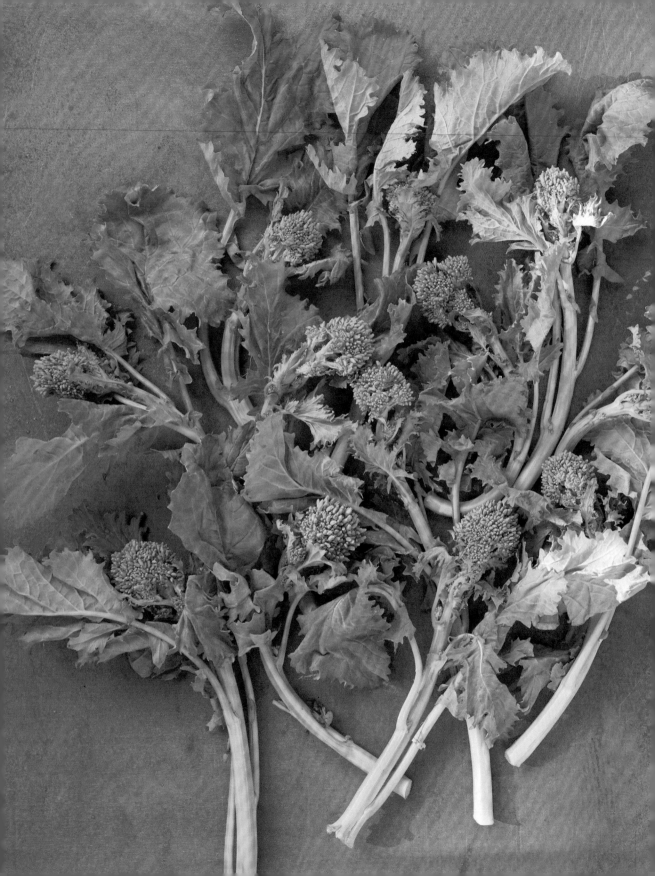

6.
PASTA and GRAIN DISHES

WHAT ITALIAN AND ASIAN COOKS DO WITH WHOLE GRAINS fascinates me as much as what they do with pasta. In Abruzzo, crisped polenta topped with broccoli rabe uses the sweetness of corn as the perfect foil for the bitter greens. But farro pasta is that region's specialty, and I learned there how this ancient form of wheat makes superb whole-grain pasta, which I use in Fusilli with Chickpeas and Tuscan Kale (p. 127).

I have not been to Asia, but learning about different varieties of rice inspired me to make pungent Kimchi Fried Rice with Crisped Tofu (p. 138) and the Black Rice Salad with Red Chard and Cranberries (p. 81) in the salad chapter.

For unexpected dishes, broccoli rabe florets paired with tortelloni gives the tender blossoms the attention they deserve. Green Fettuccini with Spinach Hemp Pesto (p. 130) is an ideal introduction to hemp seeds if you have never tried them. And the looks you will get when revealing that the crunchy bits in Quinoa Pilaf with Carrots and Kale Stems (p. 132) are the stems would make serving this whole-grain dish worthwhile even if it was not so light and colorful.

Sometimes whole-grain pasta is right for a dish. But if it is too heavy, then I prefer to use organic semolina pasta, as with creamy Baked Macaroni and Cheese with Spinach (p. 129) or big, pearl couscous in Toasted Couscous with Brussels Sprouts and Wild Mushrooms (p. 133), letting the other ingredients bring fiber and other wholesome benefits.

FUSILLI with CHICKPEAS and TUSCAN KALE

SERVES 4 |

Beans and kale ladled over dark whole-grain pasta, with the pot likker from the kale providing the moist, saucy part, make this one-pot, rustic dish positively rib-sticking. Green curly kale can be used in place of Tuscan when you Short Cook it for 4 minutes. On busy days, this is an easy go-to dinner.

8 ounces farro or whole-wheat fusilli

1 small (8-ounce) bunch Tuscan kale, stems and center veins removed

3 tablespoons extra-virgin olive oil

3 garlic cloves, smashed and peeled

½ large red onion, halved vertically and thinly sliced crosswise

1 13½- to 15½-ounce can chickpeas, drained

½ teaspoon finely chopped fresh rosemary

1 cup fat-free reduced-sodium chicken broth

Salt and freshly ground pepper

3 tablespoons grated Pecorino Romano cheese

FARRO PASTA

Farro pasta from Italy tastes nicely nutty, without the bitter taste some pastas have. Rustichella d'Abruzzo and Latini are my favorite brands. They are made using brass dies that help them hold sauces better. If it seems expensive, think of it as your protein—compared to the price of meat or poultry, it is reasonable.

---

1. In a large pot of boiling water, cook the pasta according to package directions. Drain the pasta in a colander and set aside.

2. In a large covered saucepan, boil 6 cups of water over high heat. Add the kale, pushing it into the water with a wooden spoon. Cook until the kale is very tender, 6 minutes. Ladle out and reserve 1 cup of the cooking water, then drain the kale in a colander. Run cold water over the kale while swishing with your hand until it feels cool, 30 seconds. Gather the kale and squeeze it to remove excess water. Chop the kale and pull it apart; there will be about 1¼ cups. Discard the rest of the cooking water.

3. In the pot used to cook the kale, heat the olive oil over medium-high heat. Add the garlic and cook until it is lightly browned, about 4 minutes. Remove the garlic and discard. Add the onion and cook, stirring occasionally, until it is limp, 2 minutes. Add the kale, chickpeas, rosemary, and broth, and simmer until the kale is tender, 10 minutes, stirring occasionally. Season with salt and pepper.

4. To serve, divide the fusilli among four pasta bowls. Spoon one-fourth of the kale topping and reserved liquid from the pot over the pasta. Sprinkle on the cheese.

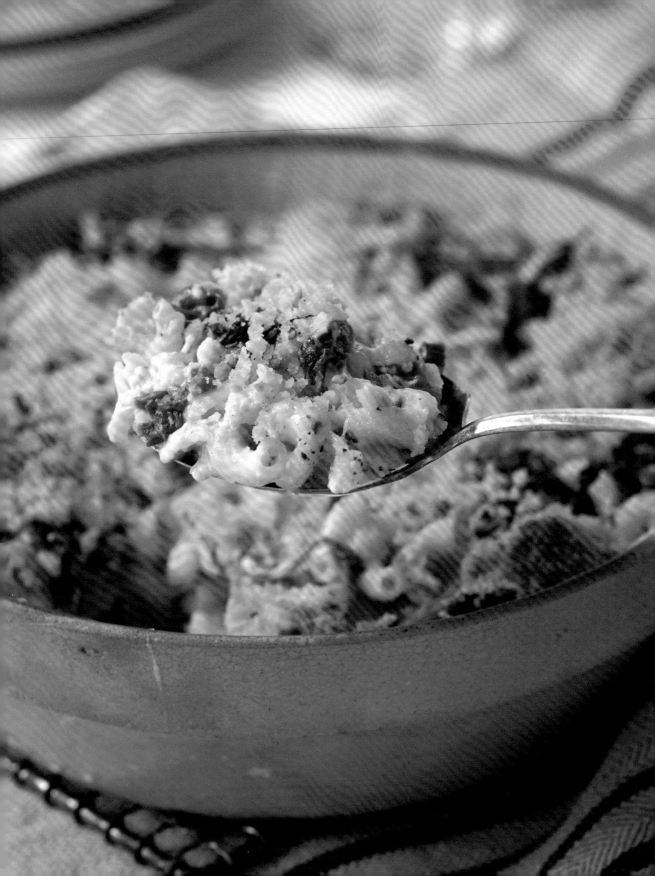

BAKED MACARONI and CHEESE with SPINACH

SERVES 4 |

You make this creamy mac and cheese by layering the pasta and cheese in a baking dish, then adding a mixture of milk and eggs. It feels simple since you don't have to make a white sauce or scrub out a cheese-encrusted pot. This dish is equally enjoyable made with whole-fat milk and cheese or using the lower-fat versions, while the eggs bring extra protein.

½ pound elbow macaroni or fusilli semolina pasta

2¼ cups whole or reduced-fat 2% milk

2 large eggs

½ teaspoon paprika

Pinch freshly grated nutmeg

1 teaspoon salt

Freshly ground pepper

Cayenne pepper

1 10-ounce package frozen chopped spinach, defrosted and squeezed dry

8 ounces shredded sharp Cheddar cheese, regular or light (2 cups)

½ cup panko crumbs

2 teaspoons extra-virgin olive oil

ANOTHER WAY

Use Short Cooked collard greens, kale, or broccoli leaf instead of spinach if you want to add cruciferous benefits. For the cheese, using a combination of Fontina cheese and Cheddar complements the stronger taste of these greens.

1. Preheat the oven to 350°F. Coat a 7 × 11-inch baking dish with cooking spray and set aside. Boil a large pot of salted water.

2. Cook the pasta according to package directions, leaving it al dente. Drain the pasta in a colander.

3. Meanwhile, in a medium saucepan, heat the milk until bubbles start to form around the edge; do not boil. Remove from the heat and whisk in the eggs, paprika, nutmeg, salt, 4 grinds of pepper, and a dash of cayenne.

4. In the prepared baking dish, spread half the pasta in an even layer. Sprinkle half the spinach over the pasta, then add half the shredded cheese. Repeat, making a second layer. Pour the milk mixture over the casserole. Cover the baking dish with foil.

5. Bake for 25 to 30 minutes. Meanwhile, in a small bowl, combine the panko and oil, working them with your fingers to coat the crumbs. Uncover the baked pasta and sprinkle the panko evenly over it. Return to the oven and bake, uncovered, for 15 minutes or until the breadcrumbs are golden. Let set for 10 minutes before serving.

GREEN FETTUCCINI with SPINACH HEMP PESTO

SERVES 4 |

When I stick to eating foods in season, my body reminds me how right this feels. So in summer, my pesto uses basil by the armload. During the cold months, I prefer this more robust version using mostly spinach. One day, lacking enough almonds, I included hemp seeds and liked the earthy note and creaminess they added. The darker flavor of this pesto fits the mood of cooler days as well as making better sense for cost through the winter when basil, often hothouse grown, comes only in modest bunches.

3 firmly packed cups stemmed flat-leaf spinach

6 large basil leaves, torn into 3 or 4 pieces

2 garlic cloves, coarsely chopped

⅓ cup slivered almonds

3 tablespoons shelled hemp seeds

1 teaspoon salt

Freshly ground pepper

¼ cup mildly grassy extra-virgin olive oil, such as Mahjoub or Kirkland organic

12 ounces spinach fettuccini, fresh or dried

1. For the pesto, in a food processor, pulse the spinach, basil, garlic, almonds, hemp seeds, salt, and 4 grinds of pepper until the mixture looks moist, 20 to 25 times. With the motor running, drizzle in the oil, and continue to whirl the pesto for 1 minute, until it is thick, with a grainy texture, scraping down the sides of the bowl once or twice. There will be nearly 1 cup pesto.

2. In a large pot of boiling water, cook the pasta following package directions. Reserve ½ cup of the pasta water, then drain the fettuccini in a colander. Divide the pasta among four pasta bowls. Top each serving with one-fourth of the pesto. Add 1 or 2 tablespoons of the reserved pasta water and toss until the pasta is covered with the pesto. Serve immediately.

HEMP SEEDS

Shelled raw hemp seeds look like hulled sesame seeds. A triple-header nutritionally speaking, they contain anti-inflammatory omega-3s, are rich in complete protein, and are an excellent source of many minerals. Buy them in a bag or loose, in bulk, at natural food stores. Their nutty flavor also goes well sprinkled on salads and in smoothies.

TORTELLONI with BROCCOLI RABE FLORETS

SERVES 4 AS A PASTA COURSE, 3 AS A MAIN DISH |

Simple yet elegant, this dish is ideal as a dinner party first course. Cooking the tender florets on their own lets you keep them crisp-tender. Then short-cook the rest of the bunch and use it to make Twice-Baked Potato with Broccoli Rabe (p. 205) or Italian Braised Greens with Roasted Garlic (p. 145) to serve another day. Chicken ravioli or spinach-and-cheese-filled tortellini are also good to use.

Florets from 1 bunch broccoli rabe (1 to 2 cups)

1 10-ounce package fresh tortelloni with cheese or pesto filling

¼ cup extra-virgin olive oil

3 garlic cloves, sliced

½ cup coarsely shredded Parmigiano-Reggiano cheese (about 2 ounces)

Freshly ground pepper

1. Fill a pasta pot halfway with water, cover, and boil over high heat. Cook the broccoli rabe florets in the boiling water for 1 minute. Using a skimmer, transfer them to a bowl and cool the florets under cold running water. Drain the rabe florets in a colander.

2. Return the water in the pot to a boil. Cook the tortelloni according to package directions. Drain the pasta, reserving ½ cup of the cooking water.

3. Meanwhile, in a large skillet, heat the oil over medium-high heat. Cook the garlic until it is golden on both sides, 4 to 5 minutes. Remove and discard the garlic. Add the rabe florets to the garlic-infused oil, stirring with a wooden spoon to coat them. Add the tortelloni and reserved cooking water, reheating the pasta for 2 minutes. If it sticks a little, nudge the pasta with the spoon. Add 4 grinds of pepper.

4. To serve, divide the pasta among four pasta bowls and sprinkle on the cheese.

DATE NIGHT DINNER

For a decadent dinner for two, in place of olive oil, melt 6 tablespoons of unsalted butter in a skillet over low heat until it browns, 10 minutes. Skim off the foam, mash in 3 roasted garlic cloves, and spoon the butter over the pasta and rabe florets. Serve with a chilled Soave. Add chocolate-dipped strawberries for dessert and who knows what may follow!

QUINOA PILAF with CARROT and KALE STEMS

SERVES 4 |

Toast quinoa, and the grains will triple in size as they cook, making an exquisitely light pilaf. Tossing the quinoa with chopped carrot and kale stems brings color, crunch, and the fun of telling guests they are eating kale stems. Serve with Indian Greens with Lemon Dal (p. 93). Vegans can use vegetable broth, which will turn the quinoa slightly orange.

¾ cup fat-free reduced-sodium chicken broth, or vegetable broth

½ cup golden quinoa

1 tablespoon extra-virgin olive oil

½ small carrot, finely chopped (2 tablespoons)

⅓ cup kale stems, thinly sliced

⅓ cup finely chopped red onion

Salt and freshly ground pepper

1. Combine the broth with ¾ cup water.

2. Rinse the quinoa in a fine-mesh strainer under cold running water.

3. In a heavy medium saucepan, toast the damp quinoa over medium-high heat, stirring frequently, until it smells fragrant and the grains start to crackle and pop, 5 minutes. Off the heat, pour in the liquid, standing back, as it will spatter. Return the pot to the heat, cover, and simmer until the quinoa is fluffy and tender, 15 minutes. Let the covered quinoa sit for 10 minutes. Season with salt and pepper.

4. While the quinoa cooks, in a medium skillet, heat the oil over medium-high heat. Add the carrot, kale stems, and onion, and cook, stirring occasionally, until the onion is translucent, 4 minutes. Add the quinoa, gently mixing to combine it with the vegetables. Serve hot or warm.

NUTRINOTE

The protein in quinoa makes it ideal to serve with meatless curries instead of rice. This pilaf is also a great gluten-free replacement for couscous.

WHAT ARE THE CURLY BITS?

The curved white bits clinging to the lid and the sides of the pot are the germ from the quinoa. They separate as the quinoa cooks. Add them to the skillet along with the grain.

TOASTED COUSCOUS with BRUSSELS SPROUTS and WILD MUSHROOMS

SERVES 4 |

Pearl couscous, aka Israeli couscous, has the texture of pasta and the lightness of more familiar, smaller-grained North African couscous. This dish has the earthy flavor of mushroom risotto. The Brussels sprouts and tomatoes add brightness and juicy contrast.

½ ounce dried wild mushrooms

1¼ cups boiling water

3 tablespoons extra virgin olive oil

1 cup pearl couscous

½ cup thinly sliced leek, white part only

6 ounces Brussels sprouts, ends removed, sliced crosswise, and separated into shreds

1 garlic clove, chopped

1 teaspoon dried thyme

2 medium plum tomatoes, seeded and chopped

Salt and freshly ground pepper

1. In a small bowl, soak the mushrooms in the boiling water until soft, 20 minutes. Strain the soaking liquid through a strainer lined with cheesecloth or a large coffee filter set over a bowl. Squeeze the soaked mushrooms, chop them, and set aside. Reserve the soaking liquid.

2. In a medium saucepan, heat 1 tablespoon of the oil over medium-high heat. Add the couscous and cook, stirring, until golden, 5 minutes. Off the heat, add the mushroom water. Return the pot to the heat, cover, and cook until the couscous is chewy-tender, 10 minutes. Set the covered couscous aside.

3. Meanwhile, in a medium skillet, heat the remaining 2 tablespoons of oil over medium-high heat. Add the leek and cook, stirring, until it is translucent, 4 minutes. Add the Brussels sprouts and garlic, and cook for 5 minutes, stirring occasionally; do not let the sprouts color. Add the chopped mushrooms and thyme. Pour in ½ cup water and cook, stirring occasionally, until the Brussels sprouts are crisp-tender and the liquid has evaporated, 7 minutes. Add the couscous and tomatoes, and cook until the pasta is heated through, 2 minutes. Season with salt and pepper, divide among 4 individual pasta bowls, and serve hot. Or serve at room temperature in a large bowl.

SEARED POLENTA with BROCCOLI RABE

SERVES 8 | (30)

Italians grill leftover polenta, then serve it with broccoli rabe. This works especially well when the broccoli rabe is cooked until creamy and soft. A generous topping of grated Parmesan cheese completes this dish as a light meal. Serving it with a platter of Italian *salume* is sympatico when you want a heartier dinner. Make the polenta ahead and you have dinner in less than thirty minutes. Vegans can skip the cheese.

1 recipe Baked Polenta (p. 136)

1 tablespoon extra-virgin olive oil, plus more as needed

2 bunches broccoli rabe, cooked as Italian Braised Greens with Roasted Garlic (p. 145)

Grated Parmesan cheese, optional

1. Cut the polenta into 4 squares. Halve each square horizontally, making 8 pieces.

2. To sear the polenta, in a large skillet, heat the oil over medium-high heat. Add the polenta and cook until it is golden and crisp on the bottom, 4 to 5 minutes. Turn and crisp on the second side, 4 minutes. You will have to do this in two batches. Or, brush the polenta with the oil and grill it in a heated grill pan until the pieces are well marked, 3 to 4 minutes on each side. Cut each piece into 2 triangles.

3. To serve, divide the broccoli rabe among eight plates. Top each serving with two polenta triangles. If desired, pass grated Parmesan cheese on the side.

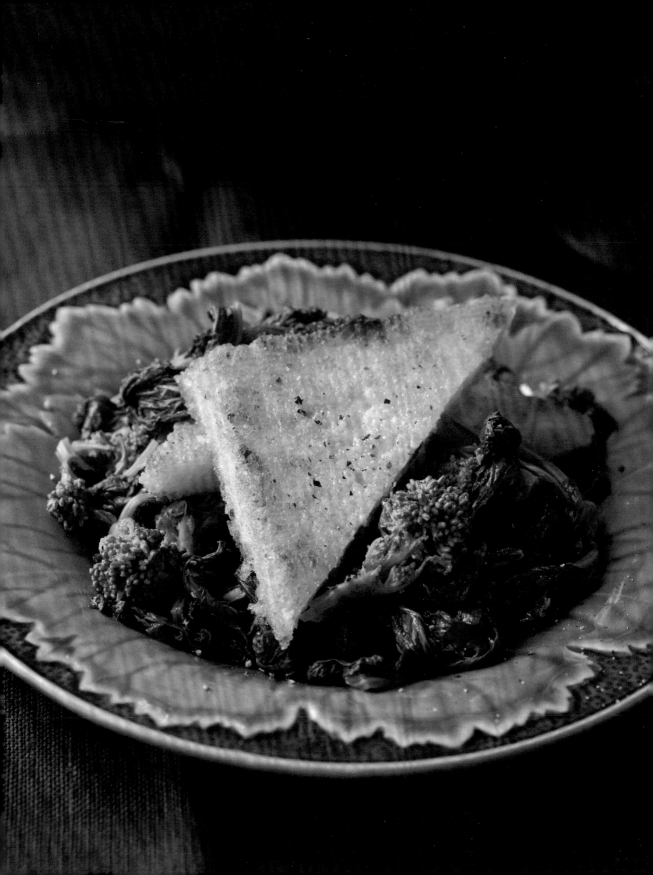

BAKED POLENTA

SERVES 4 |

Blend creamy baked polenta with grated Parmigiano cheese and serve it immediately, or let cool to make Seared Polenta with Broccoli Rabe (p. 000), using broccoli rabe cooked as in the Italian Braised Greens technique (p. 145). While the polenta bakes, you can make the greens. I like using Bob's Red Mill Polenta for its rustic, not-quite-creamy texture.

1 cup polenta or stone-ground yellow cornmeal

1 tablespoon extra-virgin olive oil

4 cups boiling water

½ teaspoon salt

1. Place a rack in the center of the oven. Preheat the oven to 350°F.

2. In a medium Dutch oven or other ovenproof pot, stir the cornmeal and oil together. Cook over medium heat, stirring until the cornmeal feels hot to the touch, about 3 minutes. Off the heat, pour in 1 cup of the boiling water, standing back, as it will spatter. Add the rest of the hot water and stir for 1 minute. Add the salt.

3. Place the polenta in the oven and bake, uncovered, for 20 minutes. Stir for 30 seconds. Bake the polenta for 20 more minutes. Mix in the crust on top and bake until the polenta is thick and creamy, about 10 minutes more.

4. Meanwhile, rinse a 9-inch square baking dish with cold water. Drain but do not dry the dish. Spoon the polenta into the wet dish, smoothing the top. Cover the polenta with plastic wrap, pressing it onto the surface so a skin does not form. Cool the polenta to room temperature.

To store: Refrigerate the cooled polenta in the pan or un-molded on a plate and covered for up to 3 days.

ANOTHER WAY

Instead of pan-crisping, you can reheat sliced polenta in foil in a 350°F oven, or grill it.

INCENDIARY HERBED BROWN RICE

SERVES 4 TO 6 |

Friends call this pilaf diabolical since no visual cue tells you that it will ignite your tastebuds. Chiles pureed in the cooking water are the secret of its invisible heat. Fresh herbs in the cooking liquid add flavor that complements this fire. They also tint the rice a soft green. When serving this dish, it is up to you whether to let guests know or to surprise them.

1 or 2 serrano chile peppers

1 small onion, diced

1 garlic clove, halved

8 to 10 cilantro sprigs, lower stems removed

6 to 8 flat-leaf parsley sprigs

1 teaspoon salt

¾ cup long-grain brown rice

1. Spear the pepper on a fork and hold it over an open flame until the skin is blistered all over, 3 minutes. Cover the pepper in a small bowl and let it sit for 5 minutes. Using your fingers, rub off the skin. Wash your hands well, scrubbing under your nails. Coarsely chop the pepper.

2. In a medium saucepan, combine the serrano pepper, onion, garlic, cilantro, parsley, salt, and 1½ cups water. Cover, bring to a boil over medium-high heat, reduce the heat, and simmer for 10 minutes. Set aside, uncovered, to cool for 10 minutes. Whirl the contents of the saucepan in a blender until almost smooth, 1 minute.

3. In another medium saucepan, combine the rice with the pureed chile water and an additional 1½ cups water. Bring to a boil over medium-high heat, cover, reduce the heat, and simmer until the rice is tender, 45 minutes. Let the covered pot sit for 10 minutes. Fluff the cooked rice with a fork, and serve.

KIMCHI FRIED RICE with CRISPED TOFU

SERVES 4 |

Mildly hot and slightly funky, this is the lightest, fluffiest fried brown rice ever. Using Carolina's long-grain brown rice is the secret. I particularly like it garnished with cool, crunchy red radish. Skip the tofu when you want this as a side dish.

½ of a 14- to 19-ounce package firm tofu

3 tablespoons peanut oil

1 medium onion, halved and thinly sliced crosswise

1 tablespoon finely chopped ginger

2 garlic cloves, finely chopped

½ cup drained kimchi, chopped

1 teaspoon sriracha sauce, or to taste

4 cups cooked brown rice, refrigerated or frozen

2 large red radishes, finely cubed, optional, for garnish

¼ cup chopped scallion, green part only, for garnish

1. Cut the tofu vertically into three slices. Cover a baking sheet with three layers of paper towels and lay the tofu on top in one layer. Set a baking sheet on top of the tofu and weight it with two large cans of tomatoes or beans and top them with a cast-iron skillet. Make sure the baking sheet is level. Press the tofu for 10 minutes. Stack the slices and cut them into ¾-inch cubes.

2. Set a wok over high heat. When drops of water flicked into it ball up and dance, add the oil. Arrange the tofu in a single layer in the wok. When pale gold on the bottom, about 2 minutes, use tongs to turn the tofu until it is colored on three sides. Transfer the tofu to a plate and set aside.

3. In the wok, stir-fry the onion, ginger, and garlic until fragrant, 30 seconds. Add the kimchi and stir-fry for 30 seconds. Add the sriracha sauce, tofu, and rice. Stir-fry, digging deep to combine them with the kimchi mixture. When the rice looks fluffy, 2 minutes, turn it out into a serving bowl and let stand 10 minutes, uncovered.

4. Just before serving, garnish with the radishes and scallion.

COOK'S TIP

The rice must be cold or it will make a sticky mess. Use it chilled from the refrigerator, or frozen.

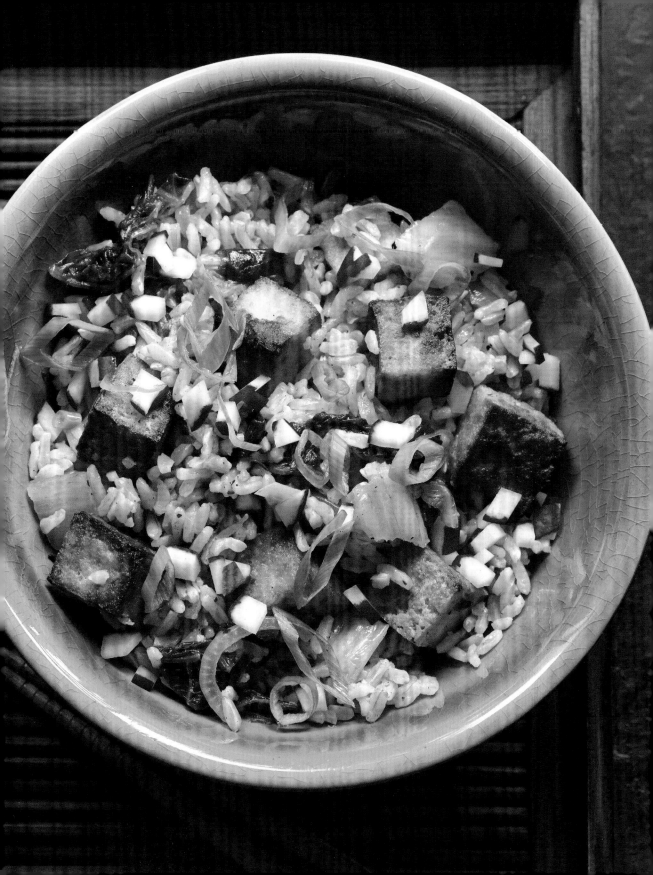

COCONUT RICE with BLACK BEANS and COLLARD GREENS

SERVES 4 |

Memories of street food are some of my favorite travel souvenirs. Perhaps the best one took place on the beach in Jamaica. I came across a man in a lean-to selling coconut rice and beans he cooked in a kettle over a charcoal fire. He pointed out a log under a nearby palm tree where I sat to eat them from a paper plate along with a pile of smoky greens. Now, I make this dish using brown rice, and with every bite, steel drums echo faintly in the background.

1 medium bunch (12 ounces) collard greens, center veins and stems removed

½ cup canned unsweetened coconut milk

1 medium onion, chopped (about 1 cup)

1 medium green pepper, seeded and chopped

¾ cup long-grain brown rice

1 medium carrot, sliced

½ cup sliced scallions, white and green parts

2 teaspoons dried thyme

¼ teaspoon ground allspice

⅛ to ¼ teaspoon red pepper flakes

1 teaspoon salt

1 15-ounce can black beans, drained

Freshly ground pepper

1. Separate each collard leaf into two long halves. Stack three or four halves and roll the leaves into a long tube. Using a sharp knife, cut the leaves crosswise into ½-inch strips.

2. In a large saucepan, bring 6 cups of water to a boil over high heat. Add the collard greens to the pot, pushing them into the water with a wooden spoon. Cook until the collards are almost tender, 6 minutes. Drain the collard greens in a colander. Run cold water over the greens while swishing with your hand until they feel cool, 30 seconds. Gather the greens together and squeeze them to remove excess water. Chop the ribbons of collard greens into bite-size pieces and then pull them apart; there will be about 2 cups.

3. In a heavy large saucepan or small Dutch oven, heat 2 tablespoons of the coconut milk over medium-high heat. Add the onion and green pepper and cook, stirring occasionally, until the onion softens, 4 minutes.

4. Mix in the rice, carrot, and the remaining coconut milk, and add 2 cups of water. Reduce the heat, and simmer, covered, for 20 minutes.

5. Add the collard greens, scallions, thyme, allspice, red pepper flakes, and 1 teaspoon salt. Cover, and simmer until the rice is tender, 20 to 25 minutes. Using a fork, mix the beans into the rice and greens. Cover, and set the pot aside

for 5 minutes to warm the beans and let the rice steam. Adjust the seasoning with salt and pepper and serve in wide, shallow pasta bowls.

___

GOOD TECHNIQUE

For Caribbean and Thai cooking, canned unsweetened full-fat coconut milk can be used for sautéing. It is a lower-fat alternative to coconut oil.

___

COOK'S TIP

Chopped green bell pepper and scallions sautéed with allspice and thyme are as quintessentially Jamaican as jerk seasoning. Toss in a can of black beans or cubed tofu for an instant, protein-rich main dish.

___

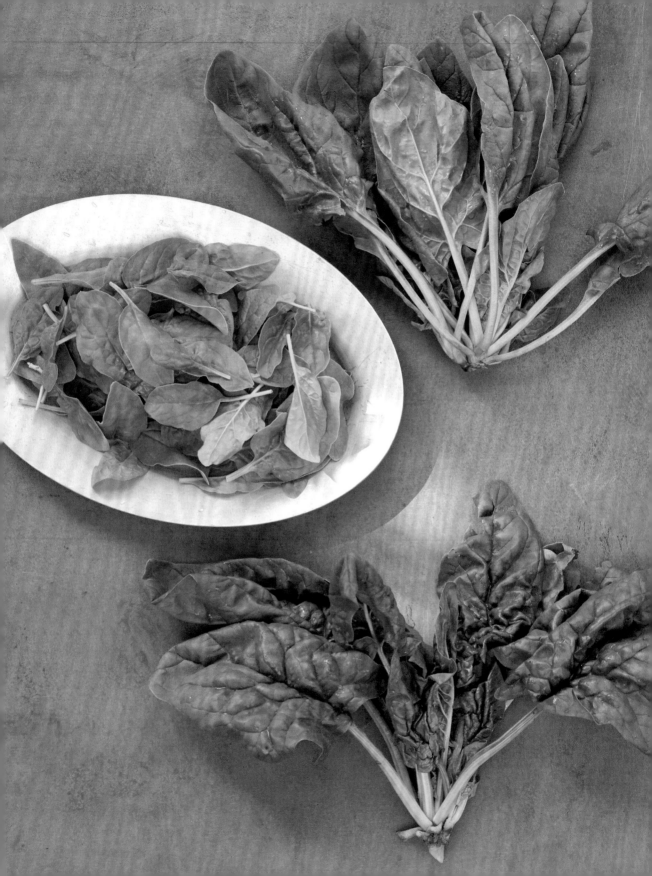

7.
SIDE DISHES and CONDIMENTS

I AM DELIGHTED THAT THE UNITED STATES HAS GONE FROM a boring carrots-and-peas nation to a land of culinary adventurers. I love the boldness and variety this calls for. Side dishes are a good place for adventurous eating, so here they include flavors from Africa and the Middle East, Mexico, and the Mediterranean, as well as regional America, and other places.

Served alongside main dishes like grilled tofu, a turkey burger, salmon, or beans and rice, they bring interest and energy while they transport you to a favorite place or introduce you to a new taste. You feel indulged while enjoying their healthy ingredients.

Virtually every Power Green gets to star in a side dish here. Some are paired with ingredients that mellow their assertive taste, like Chard with Browned Onions (p. 156), and Sweet Potato and Collard Greens Casserole (p. 163), a Southern favorite neatly including greens. Other dishes charm with their harmony, including Red Kale, Red Cabbage, and Dried Cherries (p. 171), and Broccoli Leaf, Edamame, and Corn Succotash (p. 154).

For a new experience, try creamed spinach made with tahini, Brussels sprouts in a miso-based sauce, or the fusion of stir-fried romaine lettuce with French wine. If you discover spigariello, the Italian heirloom broccoli that is leaves without florets, at the market, here's how to cook it with pancetta.

To cook dark greens in the simplest way, Italian Braised Greens with Roasted Garlic (p. 145) is a master recipe. Use it for kale, broccoli rabe, chard, spinach, and Brussels sprouts. Then enjoy variations like Tuscan Kale with Raisins and Pine Nuts (p. 149).

Finally, for bok choy, which does not appear in this chapter, serve it as a side dish using Red Chili Tofu with Baby Bok Choy (p. 100) in Main Dishes to guide you.

These recipes are detailed and precise but greens are alive and variable. Following the recipes will give delicious results but you may need to lengthen a cooking time to give a bunch of leathery greens the tenderness you prefer. Or you can use water instead of broth, as Italians do, if you want to emphasize the bitter flavor of a green. Many of these recipes use Short Cooked greens because they cut cooking times by nearly half and give you enjoyable texture.

ITALIAN BRAISED GREENS
with ROASTED GARLIC

SERVES 4 |

The way Italians cook kale, broccoli rabe, chard, or spinach with garlic and olive oil makes these pungent greens irresistible. This simple master recipe works this same magic on broccoli leaves, spigariello, or Brussels sprouts. I use roasted garlic because its caramelized flavor and creaminess mellow the bitterness of the greens while enhancing the pungent side of their taste. Short Cooking the greens before braising them reduces the total cooking time by more than half and makes them taste less sharp. Vegans can use water instead of chicken broth.

1 large bunch (16 ounces) or 2 small bunches (8 ounces each) Tuscan kale, center veins and stems removed, and torn into large pieces

2 tablespoons extra-virgin olive oil

3 or 4 large roasted garlic cloves (recipe follows)

1 cup fat-free reduced-sodium chicken broth, or water

Salt and freshly ground pepper

1. In a large covered saucepan, boil 6 cups of water over high heat. While the water boils, mound the kale on a cutting board and chop it coarsely.

2. Add the kale to the pot, pushing it into the water with a wooden spoon. Cook until it is tender, 4 minutes. Drain the kale in a colander, then run cold water over it while swishing with your hand until the kale feels cool, 30 seconds. Gather the leaves and squeeze them to remove excess water. Chop the kale and pull it apart; there will be about 3 cups.

3. In a medium skillet, heat the oil over medium-high heat. Squeeze the roasted garlic into the pan, and use a wooden spatula or spoon to mash it into the hot oil. Add the kale, mixing until it is coated with the garlic-studded oil and some garlic coats the bottom of the pan, 2 minutes. Add the liquid and simmer over medium heat, stirring occasionally, until the kale is very soft, 20 minutes. You may need to add ¼ cup of water after it has cooked for about 15 minutes. When done, the kale will be moist and the pan almost dry. Season with salt and pepper. Serve hot or luke-warm. These greens keep tightly covered in the refrigerator for 3 days. Reheat in a saucepan with just enough broth or water to be moist. Or serve at room temperature.

ROASTED GARLIC

This recipe is so useful that you should always have some in the refrigerator to use when braising greens or making pasta sauces and other dishes. It keeps for a week or longer, wrapped in foil in the refrigerator.

1 head garlic

½ teaspoon olive oil

1. Preheat the oven to 400° F.

2. Cut off the top of a head of garlic crosswise, exposing the top of all the cloves. Place the garlic on a piece of foil. Rub the head with the oil. Seal the garlic in the foil.

3. Bake until the garlic feels soft when pressed, about 45 minutes. Open the foil and let the garlic cool. To use, squeeze the head until the creamy garlic comes out of the cloves.

BRAISING OTHER GREENS

To serve 4:

Broccoli Leaf
1 bunch or bag (12 ounces): Short Cook in 6 cups water for 5 minutes. Braise for 5 to 6 minutes.

Broccoli Rabe
1 bunch (1¼ to 1½ pounds) chopped: Short Cook in 8 cups water for 6 minutes. Add the florets after 5 minutes. Braise for 20 minutes.

Brussels Sprouts
1 pound, halved vertically: Short Cook in 6 cups of water for 4 minutes. Braise for 12 to 15 minutes.

Chard
1 large (16-ounce) bunch or 2 medium (12-ounce) bunches: Short Cook in 6 cups of water for 4 minutes. Braise for 15 minutes.

Flat-Leaf Spinach
2 bunches (8 ounces each): Short Cook in 6 cups of water for 2 minutes. Braise for 10 to 12 minutes.

Curly and Tuscan Kale
1 large bunch (16 ounces): Short Cook in 6 cups of water for 4 minutes. Braise for 25 minutes.

Spigariello
2 bunches (8 ounces each): Short Cook in 6 cups of water for 6 minutes. Braise for 20 minutes.

WAYS TO USE BRAISED GREENS

Make a bed of Italian Braised Greens with Roasted Garlic (p. 145) under roast salmon or cod

Layer with Fontina cheese to make an indulgent grilled cheese sandwich

Mound on crostini or pizza

Add to a frittata

Toss with whole-grain pasta or rice, mix into polenta, or smash with potatoes

Serve with BBQ meats, cooked beans, or a roasted sweet potato

TAHINI CREAMED SPINACH

SERVES 4 |

There is luxuriously creamed spinach that contains no cholesterol and uses no compromises like skinny yogurt or fat-free sour cream. I like to make the tahini sauce by hand, but use a mini food processor if you prefer. If there are leftovers, chop and mix them into hot rice for an excellent side dish.

1 garlic clove, chopped

1 teaspoon kosher salt

½ cup tahini

½ teaspoon ground cumin

2 tablespoons fresh lemon juice

¼ to ½ cup warm water

3 tablespoons extra-virgin olive oil

2 (8-ounce) bunches flat-leaf spinach, stemmed

1. For the tahini sauce, place the garlic and salt on a cutting board, and chop until the garlic looks wet. Holding the knife blade parallel to the cutting board, use it to smear the garlic. Alternate chopping and smearing until the garlic is a rough paste, 2 minutes. Transfer the garlic to a small bowl. Add the tahini, cumin, and lemon juice, mixing to combine them. Mix in ¼ cup of the water. If the texture is too thick, continue adding water, 2 tablespoons at a time. Mix in 1 tablespoon of the oil. Set the tahini sauce aside to let its flavors meld.

2. In a large bowl of cold water, swish the spinach to shake out grit from the crevices. Transfer the spinach to a colander. Empty, rinse, and refill the bowl. Repeat until no sand or grit collects in the bottom of the bowl. Shake the spinach to get rid of excess water clinging to it.

3. In a large skillet, heat the remaining 2 tablespoons of oil over medium-high heat. Add the spinach and stir until the leaves are bright green and have collapsed, 4 minutes. Cover, and cook, until the spinach is tender, 3 to 4 minutes. Uncover, and stir until any liquid in the pan has evaporated. Transfer the spinach to a medium mixing bowl.

4. Drizzle ¼ cup of the tahini sauce over the spinach and gently mix until it coats the leaves. Add more sauce to suit your taste. Serve immediately.

COOK'S TIP

Tahini made from toasted sesame seeds tastes best. It resembles peanut butter in color.

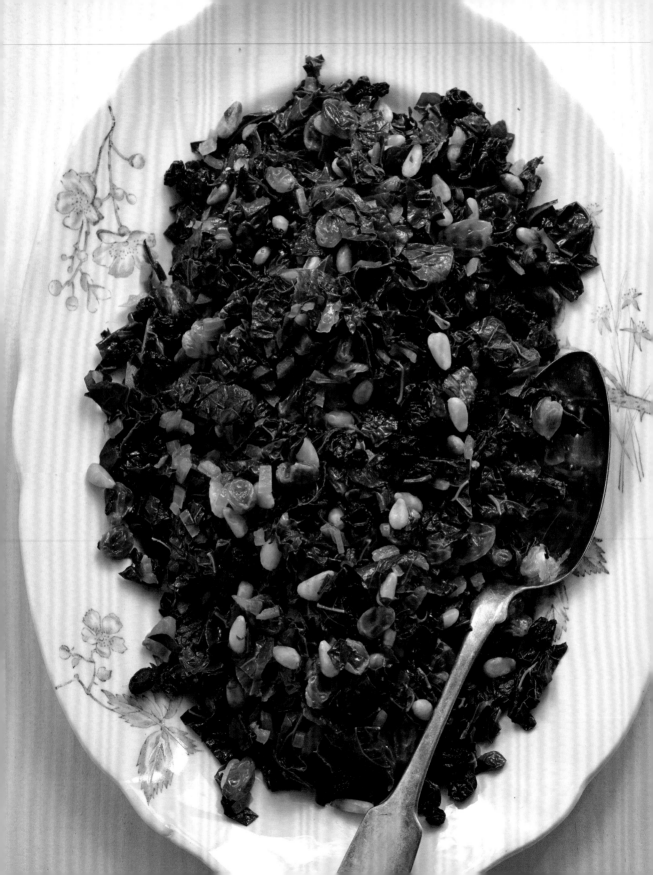

TUSCAN KALE with RAISINS and PINE NUTS

SERVES 4 |

This versatile dish can be made with any kind of kale or other greens such as spinach, chard, or broccoli rabe. Golden raisins bring a tart sweetness that goes well with greens. The anchovies add an umami lift that bolsters the overall flavor of the dish.

½ cup golden raisins

2 bunches Tuscan kale (8 to 10 ounces each), center veins and stems removed

2 tablespoons extra-virgin olive oil

1 small red onion, chopped (½ cup)

2 to 4 anchovy fillets, optional

¼ cup pine nuts

Salt and freshly ground pepper

2 tablespoons dried currants

1. In a bowl, soak the raisins in ¾ cup hot tap water until soft, 15 to 20 minutes. Drain and set aside.

2. In a covered, large saucepan, boil 8 cups of water over high heat. Add the kale, pushing it into the water with a wooden spoon. Reduce the heat to medium-high heat and cook for 6 to 8 minutes, until the kale is tender to your taste. Drain the kale in a colander, then run cold water over it while swishing with your hand until it feels cool, 30 seconds. Gather the kale and squeeze it to remove excess water. Coarsely chop the kale and pull it apart; there will be about 4 cups.

3. In a deep medium skillet, heat the oil over medium-high heat. Cook the onion, stirring occasionally, until it is golden, 6 minutes. Mash in the anchovies, if using. Stir in the kale until it looks shiny. Add the raisins, pine nuts, and 1½ cups water. Simmer, stirring occasionally, until most of the liquid has evaporated and the kale is very tender, about 15 minutes. Season with salt and pepper. Using a slotted spoon, transfer the kale to a serving bowl. Sprinkle on the currants, and serve. Leftovers keep tightly covered in the refrigerator for 3 days.

COOK'S TIP

For broccoli rabe, use 1 large bunch (1½ pounds) Short Cooked for 4 minutes before braising. Spinach and chard do not need Short Cooking.

KALE COLCANNON

SERVES 4 |

Green curly kale smashed with potatoes and smoky bacon, as the Irish combine them, is one of the best dishes I know. You can also make Colcannon using red kale, broccoli rabe, broccoli leaf, Savoy cabbage, or Brussels sprouts—simply adjust the Short Cooking and braising times to suit each green (see p. 146 for timing). Using leftover Short Cooked kale, perhaps defrosted from your freezer, works well and saves preparation time. To make it a meal, top Colcannon with a fried or poached egg.

4 medium yellow-fleshed potatoes, such as Yukon Gold (about 1 pound)

3 slices preservative-free bacon

1 medium bunch (12 ounces) green kale, center veins and stems removed

1 medium leek, white plus 1-inch light green part, halved lengthwise and sliced crosswise

Salt and freshly ground pepper

1. In a large saucepan, cover the potatoes with cold water to a depth of 3 inches. Bring to a boil, covered, over medium-high heat. Reduce the heat, and cook until a thin knife blade slips easily into the center of a potato, 25 minutes. Drain the potatoes, reserving 1 cup of the cooking water.

2. While the potatoes cook, in a medium skillet cook the bacon over medium heat until it is browned and crisp, 7 to 8 minutes. Drain the bacon on paper towels. Leave its fat in the pan.

3. Also while the bacon cooks, in a covered, large saucepan, boil 6 cups of water over high heat. Tear the kale into large pieces. Add the kale to the pot, pushing it into the water with a wooden spoon. Cover, reduce the heat to medium-high, and cook for 5 minutes, until the kale is almost tender. Drain the kale in a colander, then run cold water over it while swishing with your hand until it feels cool, 30 seconds. Gather the kale and squeeze it to remove excess water. Chop the kale and pull it apart; there will be about 1½ cups.

4. Return the skillet with the bacon fat to medium-high heat and add the sliced leek, stirring to coat it with the fat. Cook, stirring often, until the leek is limp, 4 minutes. Mix in the Quick Cooked kale, add the reserved potato water, and simmer, stirring occasionally, until the kale is tender, about 12 minutes.

5. Quarter the potatoes and add them to the skillet. Using a sturdy fork, smash and mash the potatoes and combine them with the kale until the Colcannon has the texture you like, from chunky to creamy. Off the heat, season the Colcannon with salt and pepper. Transfer the Colcannon to a serving bowl, crumble the crisp bacon over it, and serve.

To store: Leftovers keep tightly covered in the refrigerator for 2 days.

NUTRINOTE

Using unpeeled potatoes adds the good nutrients in the skin to this dish. It makes using organic potatoes a smart choice.

MUSTARD-GLAZED GREEN KALE

SERVES 4 |

Cooked greens are often livened up with a splash of vinegar. Kale tossed with sharp, whole grain mustard and a little butter tastes even better. This dish partners perfectly with pork chops or grilled tofu.

1 medium bunch green curly kale (12 ounces), center veins and stems removed

2 tablespoons unsalted sweet butter

½ teaspoon whole grain Dijon mustard

½ teaspoon fresh lemon juice

Salt and freshly ground pepper

1. In a large covered saucepan, boil 6 cups of water over high heat. Add the kale, pushing it into the water with a wooden spoon. Cook for 6 to 7 minutes, until the kale is tender. Drain in a colander, then run cold water over the kale while swishing with your hand until the greens feel cool, 30 seconds. Gather the kale and squeeze to remove excess water. Chop the kale, then pull it apart; there will be about 2 cups.

2. In a medium skillet, melt the butter over medium heat. Mix in the mustard and lemon juice. Add the kale and use tongs to turn and mix until it is coated and glistening, 2 minutes. Remove from the heat and season the kale with salt and pepper. Transfer to a serving bowl. Serve immediately.

To store: Leftovers keep tightly covered in the refrigerator for 2 days.

SPIGARIELLO with PANCETTA

SERVES 4 |

A form of broccoli resembling kale, this heirloom variety is all leaf with no florets. Braising it with a bit of pork, garlic, and tomatoes for acidity makes a rustic, truly Italian dish. Serve these tender greens with anything roasted or grilled, or toss with cooked pasta.

2 bunches spigariello (8 to 10 ounces each), center veins and stems removed, 1 large bunch Tuscan kale (16 ounces), or broccoli leaves (16 ounces)

1 tablespoon extra-virgin olive oil

3 thin slices preservative-free pancetta (about 1 ounce)

2 garlic cloves, thinly sliced

3/4 cup fat-free reduced-sodium chicken broth

2 large plum tomatoes, halved, seeded, and finely chopped

Pinch of red pepper flakes

1. In a large covered saucepan, boil 4 cups of water. Add the spigariello, pushing it into the water with a wooden spoon. Cook the spigariello for 5 minutes over medium-high heat. Drain in a colander, then run cold water over the spigariello while swishing with your hands until the greens feel cool, 30 seconds. Squeeze the spigariello to remove excess water; you may need to do this in two or more handfuls. Coarsely chop the spigariello, then pull it apart; there will be 3 to 4 cups.

2. In a medium skillet, heat the oil over medium-high heat. Add the pancetta and cook until crisp, 3 minutes, using tongs to turn it several times. Set the pancetta aside.

3. Add the garlic to the skillet. When it is golden, add the spigariello, stirring until it glistens. Add the broth plus ½ cup water, and simmer, stirring occasionally, until the greens are tender and the pan is almost dry, 15 minutes.

4. Add the tomatoes and red pepper, and cook, stirring occasionally, for 5 minutes. Transfer the spigariello to a serving bowl, crumble on the pancetta, and serve.

ANOTHER WAY

Vegans can use 2 tablespoons olive oil and 4 garlic cloves in place of the pancetta.

BROCCOLI LEAF, EDAMAME, and CORN SUCCOTASH

SERVES 4 |

Replacing this dish's customary lima beans with edamame nearly doubles the amount of protein. Broccoli leaf contributes even more, making this remarkably sustaining for a side dish. Serve it with Beets and Beet Greens with Citrus Dressing (p. 73) for a colorful, balanced vegetarian dinner. Vegans can use avocado oil or cold-pressed sesame oil.

4 large broccoli leaves, center veins and stems removed, torn into large pieces

⅓ cup finely chopped sweet onion

1 cup frozen shelled edamame

1 cup yellow corn kernels, fresh or frozen

1 large scallion, white and green parts, thinly sliced (⅓ cup)

½ cup vegetable broth or water

1 tablespoon unsalted butter

Salt and freshly ground pepper

1. In a covered, large saucepan, boil 6 cups of water over high heat. Add the broccoli leaves to the pot, pushing them into the water with a wooden spoon. Cover, reduce the heat to medium-high, and cook for 6 minutes, until the greens are tender. Drain the broccoli leaves in a colander, then run cold water over them while swishing with your hand until they feel cool, 30 seconds. Gather up the leaves and squeeze them to remove excess water. Chop the broccoli leaves and pull them apart; there will be about 1 cup.

2. In a medium saucepan, combine the onion, edamame, corn, scallion, broccoli leaves, and broth. Bring to a boil, cover, reduce the heat, and simmer until the edamame have the texture of slightly undercooked lima beans, about 5 minutes. Add the butter, stirring until it melts. Season the succotash with salt and pepper.

To store: This dish keeps covered in the refrigerator for 3 days.

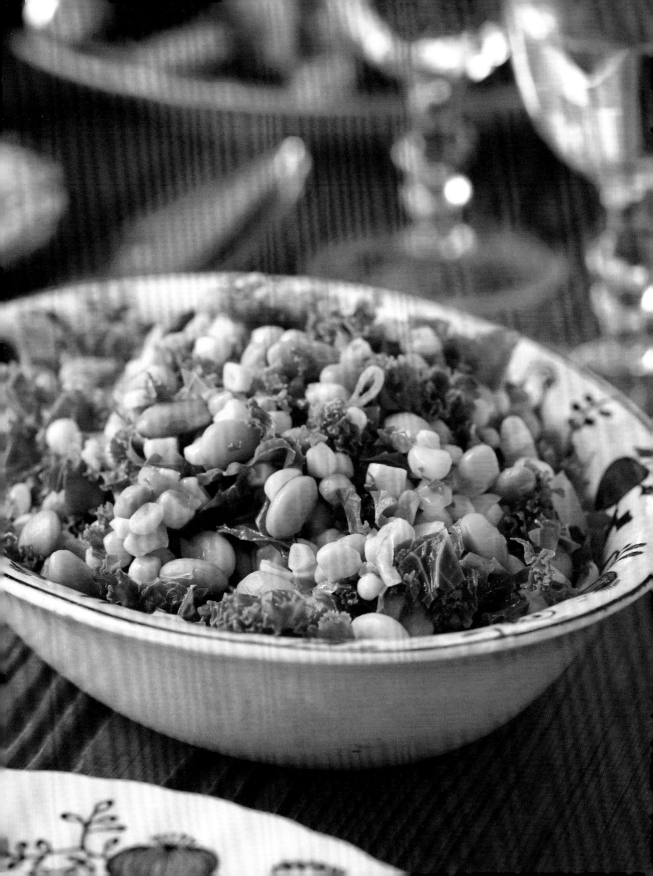

CHARD with BROWNED ONIONS

SERVES 4 |

Caramelized onion makes almost anything taste better, including mildly tannic chard. I like chard with yellow stems in this dish but green chard with white stems is fine, too. Serve this dish with everything from fried eggs at brunch to lamb chops at dinnertime.

1 bunch (12 ounces) yellow or green chard, center veins and stems removed

1 tablespoon extra-virgin olive oil

1 large onion, halved vertically and thinly sliced crosswise (about 1½ cups)

Salt and freshly ground pepper

1. To chop the chard, halve the leaves lengthwise. Stack 3 or 4 halves on a work surface with the straight center edge toward you, and roll the leaves into a long cigar. Cut the rolled chard crosswise, making strips. Gather the strips together and coarsely chop them; there will be 11 to 12 packed cups chopped chard.

2. In a medium skillet, heat the oil over medium-high heat. Add the onion, and cook, stirring occasionally, until it is translucent and limp, 5 minutes. Continue cooking the onion, stirring often, until it is browned, about 4 minutes; watch carefully so it does not burn. Transfer the onion to a plate.

3. Heap as much chard into the pan as possible. Stir with a wooden spoon to help it collapse, adding the remaining chard in handfuls. When all the chard has collapsed, 4 to 5 minutes, add ½ cup water. Cook, stirring occasionally, until the water is almost evaporated, 15 minutes. Add ¼ cup water and continue cooking, stirring more often, until the chard is tender, 10 to 15 minutes. Season with salt and pepper. Arrange the chard on a serving plate. Spoon the onion over the chard. Serve hot or warm.

To store: Leftovers keep tightly covered in the refrigerator for 3 days. Try them tossed with whole-grain pasta or mixed into cooked brown rice.

COOK'S TIPS

Short Cook the chard one or two days ahead, then warm it in a saucepan, adding a little chicken broth to prevent sticking, and stirring constantly. Top the heated chard with freshly browned onion.

ROASTED BRUSSELS SPROUTS
with MISO-ORANGE SPLASH

SERVES 4 |

Roasting caramelizes Brussels sprouts, giving them an enticing sweetness. Use either green or purple Brussels sprouts, which, unlike many other purple vegetables, hold their lovely color when cooked. You need to roast purple Brussels sprouts a bit differently, as explained, but both kinds are irresistible drizzled with this piquant miso sauce. Select Brussels sprouts that are close in size so they cook evenly.

1½ pounds green or purple Brussels sprouts, halved lengthwise

3 tablespoons avocado or olive oil

2 teaspoons mellow white miso

½ cup fresh orange juice

2 teaspoons agave syrup

Salt and freshly ground pepper

1 to 2 teaspoons grated orange zest, optional, for garnish

1. Preheat the oven to 400°F.

2. Mound the Brussels sprouts on a baking sheet, drizzle on the oil, and rub the sprouts with your hands until they are evenly coated with the oil. Spread out the Brussels sprouts in an even layer, cover loosely with foil, and roast for 12 to 15 minutes. Uncover and roast for 15 minutes longer, or until the Brussels sprouts are tender but not mushy. For purple Brussels sprouts, arrange the oiled sprouts cut-side down in one layer and roast them for 10 minutes, or until they are caramelized in places and al dente. Stir, turning over any Brussels sprouts that are getting too dark. Bake until the purple sprouts are tender but not soft, about 10 minutes.

3. Meanwhile, in a small bowl, use the back of a spoon to cream the miso with 2 tablespoons of the orange juice. Place the miso mixture in a small saucepan and add the remaining orange juice and the agave syrup. Cook over medium-high heat just until the mixture boils, 3 minutes.

4. Transfer the roasted sprouts to a serving bowl, drizzle on the miso-orange sauce, and season with salt and pepper. Garnish with the zest and serve warm or at room temperature.

COOK'S TIP

Look for purple Brussels sprouts from November through February in better supermarkets and on produce websites.

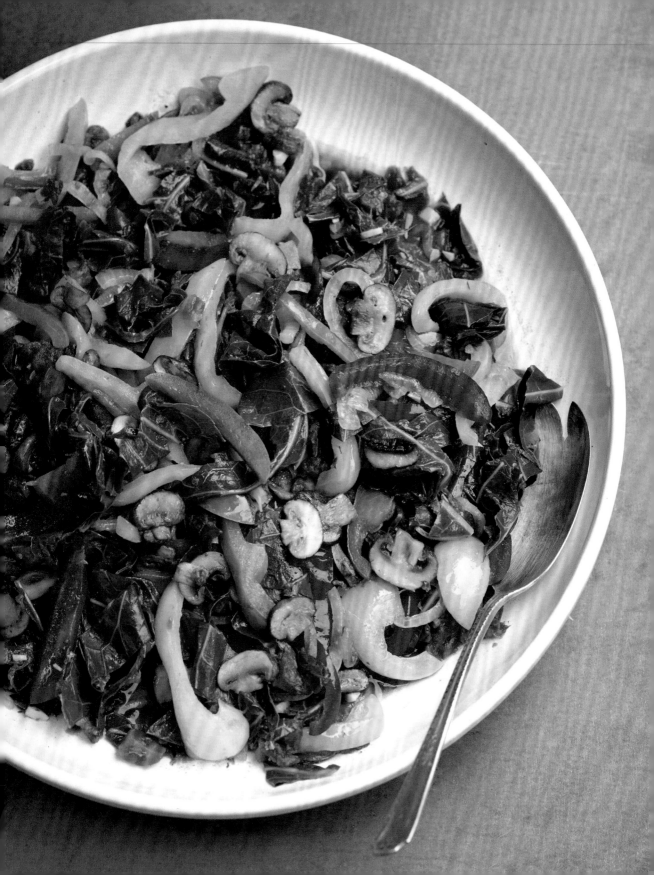

COLLARD GREENS CACCIATORE

SERVES 4 |

Mushrooms, sweet peppers, and a splash of wine turn this meatless version of a dish usually made with game into something close to a main course. The collard greens taste so mellow that I have even seen a picky four-year-old go for them. Serve accompanied by kidney beans and brown rice, alongside pan-seared pork chops or baked tilapia.

16 ounces collard greens (1 large bunch), center veins and stems removed

2 tablespoons extra-virgin olive oil

1 large onion, halved vertically and sliced crosswise

1 medium green bell pepper, seeded and cut into 1/2-inch strips

1 medium red bell pepper, seeded and cut into 1/2-inch strips

1 medium yellow bell pepper, seeded and cut into 1/2-inch strips

2 garlic cloves, chopped

1/2 pound cremini mushrooms, stemmed and sliced

1 14-ounce can diced tomatoes, preferably fire-roasted

1/2 cup white wine

2 teaspoons dried oregano

1. Halve the collard leaves lengthwise. Stack 3 or 4 halves on your work surface with their straight center edge toward you. Roll the leaves into a long cigar; if it is loose, that is fine. Cut the collards crosswise into 3/4-inch-wide strips.

2. In a covered, large saucepan, boil 8 cups of water over high heat. Add the collard greens, pushing them into the water with a wooden spoon. Cover, reduce the heat to medium-high, and cook for 8 minutes. Drain the collard greens in a colander, then run cold water over them while swishing with your hand until they feel cool, 30 seconds. Gather the greens and squeeze them to remove excess water; you may need to do this in two or more handfuls. Pull them apart; there will be about 2 1/2 cups.

3. In a deep medium skillet, heat the oil over medium-high heat. Add the onion and cook, stirring often, until it is limp, 4 minutes. Mix in the peppers and garlic, stirring until the peppers look moist, 4 minutes. Add the mushrooms and cook until they begin to release their liquid, 3 minutes. Add the collard greens, tomatoes with their liquid, wine, and oregano, and cook, uncovered, stirring 3 or 4 times, until the collards and peppers are meltingly tender, 10 minutes. Season with salt and pepper.

To store: Leftovers keep tightly covered in the refrigerator for 3 days.

ANOTHER WAY

Add thin slices of baked marinated tofu and simmer with the cacciatore until it is heated through, 5 minutes.

HASH BROWN POTATOES with COLLARD GREENS

SERVES 4 |

Creamy potatoes with crunchy bits and caramelized onion make these hash browns irresistible. The boiled potatoes have to cool before you sauté them—remember this to allow enough time for the finished dish. Serve with eggs, scrambled tofu, bacon, or a ham steak for brunch and any time you feel like having breakfast for dinner.

1 pound yellow-fleshed potatoes

3 tablespoons extra-virgin olive oil

1 medium bunch collard greens (12 ounces), center veins and stems removed

1 medium onion, finely chopped

Salt and freshly ground pepper

1. In a large saucepan, cover the potatoes with cold water to a depth of 3 inches. Cover and bring to a boil over medium-high heat. Reduce the heat and cook until a thin knife blade slips easily into the center of the potatoes, 25 minutes. Drain the potatoes. When cool enough to handle, dice the unpeeled potatoes and place them in a mixing bowl. When they are room temperature, add 1 tablespoon of the oil and toss well.

2. Meanwhile, halve the collard leaves lengthwise. Stack 3 or 4 halves on your work surface with the straight center edge toward you. Roll the leaves into a long cigar; if it is loose, that is fine. Cut the roll crosswise into ½-inch-wide strips.

3. In a large covered saucepan, boil 6 cups of water. Add the collard greens, pushing them into the water with a wooden spoon. Cover, reduce the heat to medium-high, and cook for 8 minutes. Drain the collard greens in a colander, then run cold water over them while swishing with your hand until they feel cool, 30 seconds. Gather the greens and squeeze them to remove excess water; you may need to do this in two or more handfuls. Chop the collard greens into roughly ¾-inch pieces; there will be about 1½ cups.

4. Heat the remaining 2 tablespoons oil in a large skillet, preferably cast iron, over medium-high heat. Add the onion and cook, stirring often, until it is golden, 7 minutes. Add the potatoes and cook, using a wooden spatula to scrape the bottom of the pan frequently and vigorously to gather up

the browned crust that forms. When the potatoes start to soften, add the collard greens and continue scraping and stirring until the potatoes start breaking down and are creamy, 3 or 4 minutes. Season with salt and pepper. Serve hot or lukewarm.

To store: Leftovers keep tightly covered in the refrigerator for 2 days. To reheat, wrap them in foil and place in a 350°F oven for 15 to 20 minutes.

COOK'S TIP

Using leftover cooked potatoes works splendidly. Think of this when boiling potatoes for other dishes. This dish is ready in 30 minutes.

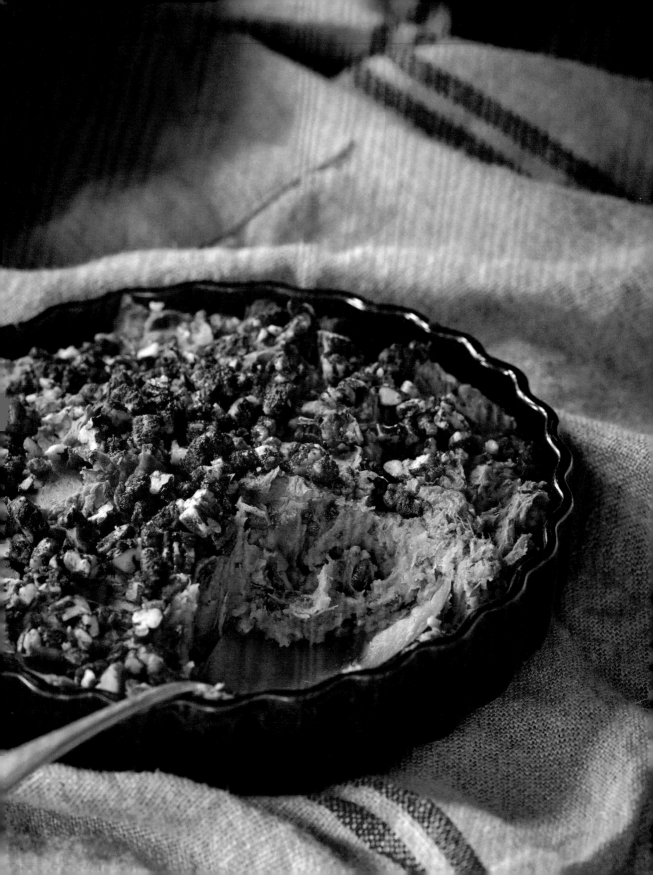

SWEET POTATO and COLLARD GREENS CASSEROLE

SERVES 6 |

I debated whether to call this a casserole or a pudding; the potatoes are so creamy that the topping could make it a not-too-sweet dessert. Using both coconut oil and coconut sugar adds a nicely nutty flavor to the topping and filling. When you feel low, this dish will make you lick the spoon and smile. Serve with turkey, pork, or tempeh, or let it be the whole meal—nutritionally, you could do far worse!

2½ pounds orange-flesh sweet potatoes, such as Garnet, Jewel, or Beauregard yams

1 small bunch collard greens (8 to 9 ounces), center veins and stems removed

1 large egg

1 tablespoon coconut sugar, or lightly packed brown sugar

1 tablespoon coconut oil

1 teaspoon grated orange zest

½ teaspoon salt

Freshly ground pepper

TOPPING

½ cup chopped pecans

2 tablespoons coconut sugar or lightly packed brown sugar

½ teaspoon ground cinnamon

1 tablespoon coconut oil

1. Preheat the oven to 400°F. Coat an 8 x 8 x 1½-inch baking dish with cooking spray.

2. Coat the sweet potatoes with cooking spray and pierce them in three places with the tip of a knife. Roast the potatoes until they are very soft when squeezed, 45 to 60 minutes. Reduce the oven temperature to 350°F.

3. While the sweet potatoes roast, halve the collard leaves lengthwise. Stack 3 or 4 halves on your work surface with their straight center edge toward you. Roll the leaves into a long cigar; if it is loose, that is fine. Cut the collards crosswise into ¾-inch strips.

4. In a covered, large saucepan, boil 8 cups of water over high heat. Add the collard greens, using a wooden spoon to push them into the water. Cover, reduce the heat to medium-high, and cook for 6 minutes. Drain the collard greens in a colander, then run cold water over them while swishing with your hand until they feel cool, 30 seconds. Gather the greens and squeeze them to remove excess water; you may need to do this in two or more handfuls. Chop the collard greens into roughly ½-inch pieces; there will be about 1½ cups.

5. When the sweet potatoes are cool enough to handle, peel them using your fingers and place the flesh in a medium mixing bowl. Break the egg into the bowl on one side, beat it lightly with a fork, then combine it with the

continued on next page

sweet potatoes, mashing them until creamy, 3 minutes. Mix in the sugar, coconut oil, zest, salt, and 4 grinds of pepper. Add the collard greens to the mashed potatoes, stirring to combine them.

6. Spread the sweet potato mixture evenly in the prepared baking dish. In a small bowl, combine the pecans, sugar, cinnamon, and coconut oil, and sprinkle the mixture evenly over the potatoes. Bake the casserole for 30 minutes, until the potatoes are heated through and the topping is crunchy. Let the casserole sit for 20 minutes before serving.

To store: Leftovers keep tightly covered in the refrigerator for 3 days.

NUTRINOTE

The fragrant compounds that give citrus zest its aroma are potent phytochemicals.

GARLIC and PARSLEY SMASHED POTATOES

SERVES 4 |

Yellow-fleshed potatoes are naturally buttery and fluffy. Mashing them with boiled garlic makes them even creamier. The result—a potato-lover's dream without a drop of fat—makes overindulging in these mashed potatoes unavoidable. Serve with roast chicken or meatloaf, top with an egg, or just eat them from the bowl. Since you eat the skins, I suggest using organic potatoes.

1 pound small yellow-fleshed potatoes, preferably organic

4 to 6 large garlic cloves, peeled

1 lightly packed cup flat-leaf parsley leaves, finely chopped

Salt and freshly ground pepper

1. In a large saucepan, cover the unpeeled potatoes and the whole garlic cloves with cold water to a depth of 2 inches. Cover, and set the pot over medium-high heat, When the water boils, reduce the heat to a gentle boil, cover, and cook until a small, sharp knife slides easily into the potatoes, about 20 minutes. Drain the potatoes and garlic in a colander.

2. Return the potatoes and garlic to the pot and place over medium heat. Shake the pot until the bottom is dry, up to 1 minute. Remove from the heat and use a sturdy fork to smash the potatoes and garlic into rough chunks. Add the parsley and mash the potatoes until they have the chunky-creamy texture you like. Season with salt and pepper. Serve immediately.

NUTRINOTE

The potato skins add good texture along with useful vitamins, minerals, and fiber.

THREE-ALARM MUSTARD GREENS

SERVES 4 |

Combining two cooking methods here, you start mustard greens as you would for a stir-fry, then add liquid and braise them until they are silky and tender. Spicy Asian seasonings, including ginger and sriracha, add even more fire to these assertively flavored greens. This dish is prepared medium-hot, but adjust the heat level to your taste.

1 large bunch mustard greens (20 ounces) or 2 medium bunches (12 ounces each)

1 tablespoon mellow white miso

2 teaspoons sriracha hot chile sauce, or to taste

½ teaspoon agave syrup

2 tablespoons vegetable broth, or water

Salt

4 teaspoons coconut oil

½-inch piece fresh ginger, cut into 4 slices

1. In a covered large saucepan, boil 8 cups of water over high heat. Tear away the tough lower portion of the mustard greens. Add the mustard greens to the pot, pushing the leaves into the water with a wooden spoon. Cover, reduce the heat to medium-high, and cook for 3 minutes, until the greens are almost tender. Drain them in a colander, then run cold water over the mustard greens while swishing with your hand until they feel cool, 30 seconds. Gather the mustard greens and squeeze them to remove excess water; this may take two or three handfuls. Chop the greens and pull them apart; there will be 4 to 5 cups.

2. In a small bowl, use the back of a wooden spoon to cream together the miso, sriracha sauce, and agave. Stir in the broth and ½ teaspoon salt.

3. In a medium skillet, heat the oil over medium-high heat. Add the ginger, and cook until the slices are just golden brown, 2 minutes, turning them a few times. Discard the ginger.

4. Add the mustard greens to the pan, stirring to coat them with the oil. Cook the greens, stirring occasionally, for 2 minutes. Add ¾ cup water, and cook, stirring occasionally, until the mustard greens are tender to your taste, 5 to 8 minutes. When the greens are almost dry, add the miso mixture, stirring to coat the greens. Adjust the salt to taste. Serve immediately.

To store: Leftovers keep tightly covered in the refrigerator for 2 days. Serve them at room temperature, the Asian way.

CHINESE CABBAGE
with PEANUT SATÉ SAUCE

SERVES 6 TO 8 |

Why use saté sauce only with meat or tofu when you can also spoon it over braised Napa, aka Chinese, cabbage? The cabbage, cooked just long enough to be tender toward the tip while remaining lightly crisp near the base, contains so much moisture that it braises mostly in its own juices. Serve with grilled flank steak, or Kimchi Fried Rice with Crisped Tofu (p. 138).

½ cup reduced-fat coconut milk

3 tablespoons smooth unsweetened peanut butter

1 tablespoon coconut sugar or packed brown sugar

½ teaspoon garlic powder

2 teaspoons reduced-sodium soy sauce

2 teaspoons fresh lime juice

¼ to ½ teaspoon red pepper flakes

½ teaspoon salt

⅛ teaspoon freshly ground pepper

1 small head Napa cabbage, 1¾ to 2 pounds

2 tablespoons peanut oil

⅓ cup fat-free reduced-sodium chicken broth

1. In a small saucepan, mix together the coconut milk, peanut butter, sugar, garlic powder, soy sauce, lime juice, pepper flakes, salt, and ground pepper until the sauce is smooth. Cook the sauce over medium-high heat just until it boils. Stir and set the sauce aside.

2. Cut the head of cabbage in half lengthwise. Cut each half into 3 or 4 long wedges, depending on the size of the cabbage.

3. Heat the oil in a large skillet over medium-high heat. Arrange the cabbage in the pan, fitting the wedges together tightly and alternating the direction in which the tips point. Place wedges across the top and bottom of the aligned ones, if necessary. Cook until the cabbage is browned in places, 2 minutes. Using tongs, turn the wedges, end over end, pour in the broth, cover, and cook until the cabbage is translucent and tender-crisp, 5 minutes. Transfer each wedge to a plate alongside the main course, or set on top of cooked rice. Season the sauce to taste with salt, spoon the sauce over the cabbage, and serve.

To store: Leftover sauce keeps covered in the refrigerator for 3 days. Leftover cabbage will be too mushy to serve but it is good chopped up and added to a vegetable soup.

ROASTED CABBAGE DRIZZLED with GREEN HARISSA

SERVES 4 TO 6 |

Roasted cabbage is moist and tender but not limp. Pairing it with harissa occurred to me when I needed to dress up this dish for company. Cumin and fennel add complexity to the harissa's heat. Fresh herbs add even more flavor to this Mediterranean hot stuff. Although not the most colorful dish, the combination of spicy harissa against the caramelized sweetness of the cabbage makes it a keeper.

FOR THE HARISSA

1 large jalapeño pepper

½ cup firmly packed cilantro leaves

½ cup firmly packed flat-leaf parsley leaves

1 garlic clove, chopped

½ teaspoon ground cumin

¼ teaspoon ground fennel or ½ teaspoon fennel seed

¼ teaspoon salt

½ teaspoon fresh lemon juice

⅓ cup extra-virgin olive oil

· · · · · ·

1 medium Savoy or red cabbage (about 2 pounds)

3-4 tablespoons extra-virgin olive oil

Sea salt

1. Preheat the oven to 400°F. Line a baking sheet with foil and set it aside.

2. Over an open flame, roast the jalapeño until its skin is blistered, 2 to 3 minutes. Place the jalapeño in a small bowl, cover, and let it steam for 10 minutes. With your fingers, slip off the blistered skin. Seed the pepper, or leave some or all of the seeds and ribs, depending on how hot you want the harissa to be. Coarsely chop the pepper.

3. In a mini food processor, whirl the cilantro, parsley, garlic, cumin, fennel, and salt until the herbs are finely chopped, 1 minute. Add the jalapeño and lemon juice, then, with the motor running, drizzle in the oil. Transfer the harissa to a small bowl or glass jar, cover, and let sit for 30 minutes to let the flavors develop and meld.

4. Halve the cabbage vertically and discard the tough outer layers. Cut each half vertically into 4 wedges, including part of the core to hold the leaves together. Arrange the cabbage wedges on the prepared baking sheet, leaving ½ inch between them. Brush the cabbage generously with the oil on all sides. Season the wedges with a pinch of salt.

5. Roast the cabbage for 15 minutes. Using tongs, turn the wedges. Brush the cabbage again with oil and season with salt. Bake until the cabbage is soft but not collapsing, 15 to 20 minutes. Cool the cabbage on the baking sheet until

Continued on page 170

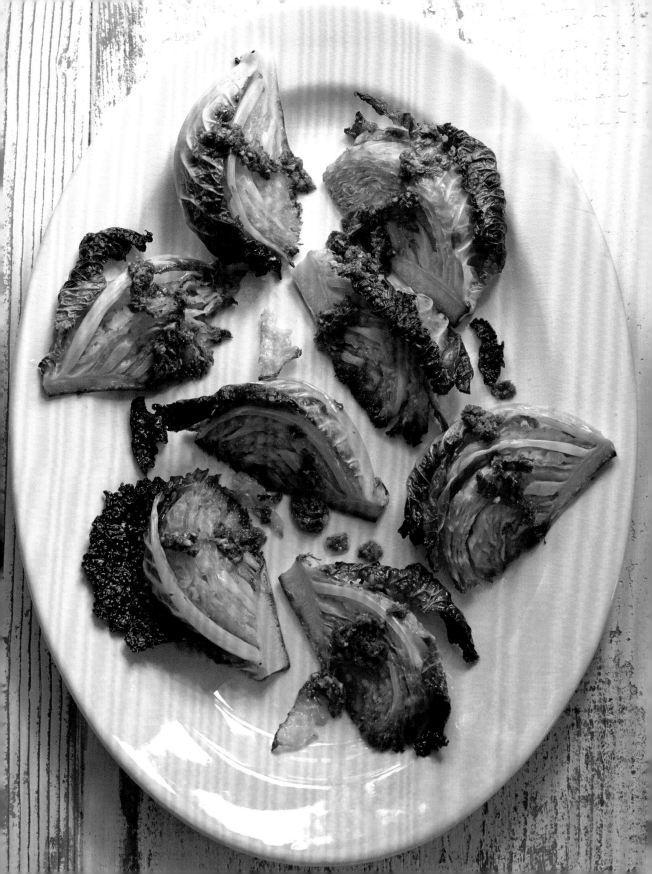

lukewarm. Arrange the cabbage on a platter. Drizzle on the harissa and serve.

To store: Leftovers keep tightly covered in the refrigerator for 2 days. Serve them at room temperature, like a Moroccan salad. Extra harissa keeps for up to 3 days, tightly covered in the refrigerator.

COOK'S TIP

Savoy and red cabbage contain more sugar than green cabbage, which helps them caramelize easily when roasted.

USE IT WITH

Green Harissa can be a dip served with pita chips. It also goes with other steamed or roasted vegetables, grilled meat, poultry, seafood, tofu, and eggs. Dollop it into soups, mix it with mayo to use on sandwiches, and try it in tuna salad. Of course it is great with couscous and with beans or rice, too.

RED KALE, RED CABBAGE, and DRIED CHERRIES

SERVES 4 |

Braising melds together the tender kale and firmer cabbage in this sweet and sour dish. Pomegranate juice and dried cherries bring enough sweet and tart flavors that you need a minimal amount of added sugar and vinegar. Serve with pan-seared turkey cutlets, lean pork chops, or grilled tempeh. It is also perfect with sauerbraten.

1 small bunch (8 ounces) red Russian kale, stemmed

2 tablespoons canola oil

1 cup red onion cut into thin crescents

4 cups finely shredded red cabbage

⅓ cup dried sour cherries

1 tablespoon packed brown sugar

¼ teaspoon ground ginger

1 cup pomegranate juice

1 tablespoon balsamic vinegar

1 teaspoon salt

Freshly ground pepper

1. In a covered, large saucepan, boil 8 cups of water over high heat. Add the kale, pushing it into the water with a wooden spoon. Cover, reduce the heat to medium-high, and cook for 5 minutes. Drain the kale in a colander, then run cold water over it while swishing with your hand until it feels cool, 30 seconds. Gather the leaves and squeeze them to remove excess water. Chop the kale and pull it apart; there will be about 1 cup.

2. In a deep medium skillet with a cover, heat the oil over medium-high heat. Add the onion and cabbage. Stir until the cabbage collapses, 5 minutes. Cover, reduce the heat to medium-low, and cook until the cabbage and onion are very moist, 4 minutes.

3. Add the kale, cherries, sugar, ginger, pomegranate juice, vinegar, and salt, plus 5 or 6 grinds of pepper. Mix and spread the vegetables in an even layer. Cover and simmer gently for 20 minutes, adjusting the heat as needed. Uncover, and cook until the cabbage and onion are meltingly tender and the liquid is nearly evaporated, 10 minutes, stirring frequently. Serve almost hot, or warm.

To store: Leftovers keep tightly covered in the refrigerator for 4 days.

NUTRINOTE

Ground ginger provides the same anti-inflammatory benefits as fresh ginger.

FRENCH LETTUCE STIR-FRY

SERVES 4 |

When the French braise lettuce, an unexpected nutty flavor emerges. Stir-frying also brings out this flavor while keeping the crunch that makes romaine popular. Fusing French ingredients with Chinese technique, this side dish is good accompanying salmon, roasted white fish like branzino or trout, or grilled tofu.

1 tablespoon dry vermouth

1 teaspoon reduced-sodium soy sauce

3/4 teaspoon salt

1/2 teaspoon sugar

1 tablespoon avocado oil or light olive oil

2 large shallots, thinly sliced vertically

1 large head romaine lettuce, about 1 pound, cut crosswise into 1-inch strips

1. In a small bowl, combine the vermouth, soy sauce, salt, and sugar, stirring until the sugar and salt dissolve.

2. Set a wok over high heat. When drops of water flicked into the wok ball up and dance, swirl in the oil. Add the shallots and stir-fry until they look translucent, 30 seconds. Add all the lettuce at once and stir-fry until it is coated with oil and bright green, 1 minute. Restir and pour in the seasoning sauce. Stir-fry until the soft parts of the lettuce are dark green and the spines are translucent and crisp, 1 to 2 minutes. Transfer the lettuce to a serving dish and serve immediately.

COOK'S TIPS

Avocado oil has a high smoke point suited to stir-frying and a light flavor good with lettuce.

If the shallots char a bit, it will just add to the dish's flavor.

USING UMAMI

Long before umami was named the fifth flavor, I worked with a chef who snuck a drop of soy sauce into his *beurre blanc*. No one could figure out why his version of this butter sauce tasted so mouth-filling. By bringing umami, the soy sauce here has the same effect.

CARROTS with WILD ARUGULA PESTO

SERVES 4 |

Carrots go particularly well with this dairy-free, nutty pesto. They are so good together that I often double the recipe to enjoy this carotene-rich dish warm, and then again at room temperature. For a colorful antipasto, serve this sunny dish together with Roasted Red Peppers Stuffed with Kale (p. 31) and Caponata of Dark Greens (p. 26).

3 large carrots, cut diagonally into ½-inch slices

Wild Arugula Pesto (p. 175)

1 teaspoon fresh lime juice

1 teaspoon extra-virgin olive oil

Salt and freshly ground pepper

1. Set a steamer basket into a large saucepan and add 1 inch of water. Cover and bring the water to a boil over medium-high heat. Add the carrots and steam, covered, for 5 minutes. Transfer the carrots to a serving bowl.

2. Add the pesto, lime juice, and olive oil to the carrots, using a fork to toss gently until the carrots are coated. Season with salt and pepper. Serve warm or at room temperature.

COOK'S TIP

The big, fat carrots sold loose for juicing are often the sweetest, making them ideal for this dish.

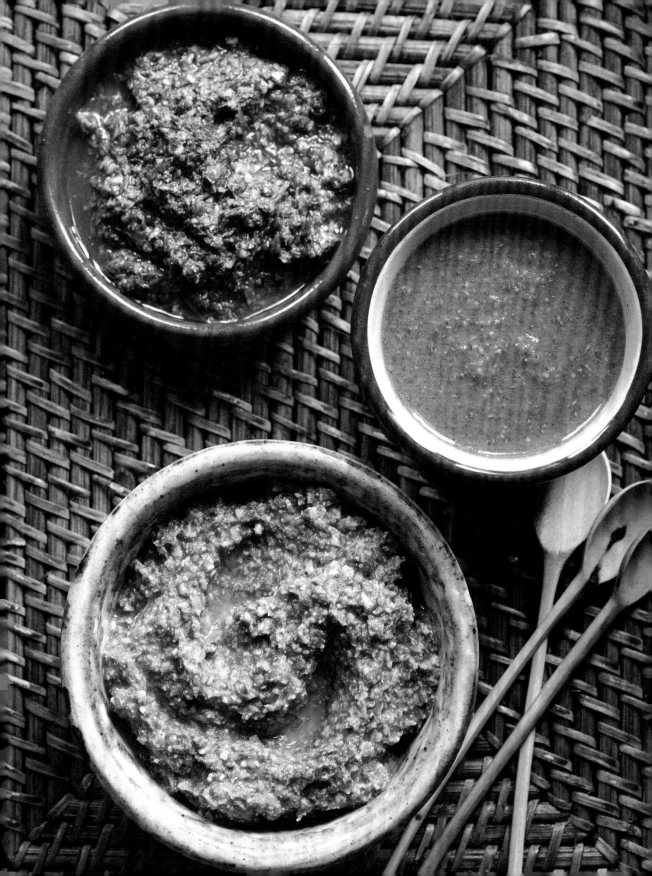

WILD ARUGULA PESTO

MAKES 7/8 CUP |

Wild arugula is potent but it does not dominate like basil, so you can taste the sweetness of the pistachios and bite of the shallot along with its sharpness. This condiment enhances the flavor of so much more than pasta. You will also want to use it on vegetables from artichokes to zucchini—tossing it with steamed carrots is just one example (see p. 173). Also serve it with an omelet, beans, grains, and seafood, including shrimp, salmon, roasted white fish like branzino or trout, and grilled tofu.

3 packed cups wild arugula

1 large shallot, chopped (about 2 tablespoons)

⅓ cup shelled pistachios

⅓ cup extra-virgin olive oil, preferably a fruity one

1 teaspoon fresh lemon juice

Salt and freshly ground pepper

In a food processor, combine the arugula and shallot and whirl until finely chopped. Add the nuts and whirl until the arugula looks moist, about 1 minute. With the motor running, drizzle in the oil, then the lemon juice. Season with salt and pepper. This pesto keeps tightly covered in the refrigerator for 3 days.

ANOTHER WAY

For a variation using regular arugula, almonds, and garlic, see Grilled Eggplant Stacks with Red Pepper, Mozzarella, and Arugula Pesto (p. 97)

TOP TO BOTTOM:

Green Harissa, Red Chimichurri,

and Arugula Pesto

RED CHIMICHURRI

MAKES 3/4 CUP |

Vinegar in this pungent South American condiment makes it perfect to serve with grilled beef. In Marical Prescilla's compendium of Latin American food, *Gran Cocina Latina,* I found a gentler, citrus-sparked version of this table sauce that goes well with other foods, too. Blending the flavors of onion, cilantro, Spanish paprika, fresh herbs, and lemon juice, it is so good you want to slurp it from a spoon. It livens up grilled chicken and pan-seared turkey cutlets, as well as grass-fed burgers, flank steak, or even a pork tenderloin.

½ cup chopped red onion

¼ firmly packed cup cilantro

4 garlic cloves, coarsely chopped

1½ teaspoons dried oregano

1½ teaspoons sweet Spanish paprika

¼ teaspoon cayenne pepper, optional

¼ cup fresh lemon juice

¼ cup extra-virgin olive oil

Salt and freshly ground pepper

Combine the onion, cilantro, garlic, oregano, paprika, and cayenne, if using, in a food processor and pulse until they are coarsely chopped. Add the lemon juice and oil, and pulse until they are combined. Season with salt and pepper. This condiment keeps tightly covered in the refrigerator for 5 days.

COOK'S TIP

For a salad with a kick, toss romaine lettuce, sliced cucumber, and red onion rings with Red Chimichurri.

KALE ZA'ATAR

MAKES 1/3 CUP |

Za'atar, an herb that tastes somewhere between thyme, oregano, and marjoram, grows wild around the eastern end of the Mediterranean. Za'atar is also a seasoning made by combining the herb za'atar with sesame seeds, sumac, and salt. Since the herb za'atar is seldom available, here I use thyme in its place. Adding crushed Crisped Kale enhances the nutty side of this condiment. Use Za'atar to make a two-part dip by first dunking bread or pita chips into a bowl of olive oil and then a bowl of za'atar. Its flavor goes well with hummus, avocado toast, lentils, navy beans, cooked rice, and even quinoa. Sprinkle it, too, on yogurt, cottage cheese, grilled fish, or oatmeal (really).

1 cup Crisped Kale (p. 178)

1 tablespoon fresh thyme leaves

1½ teaspoons sumac

¼ teaspoon salt, optional

3 tablespoons sesame seeds

1. Place the kale in a mixing bowl and crush it finely with your fingers, removing any long strawlike pieces. Add the thyme leaves, sumac, and salt, if using.

2. In a small, dry skillet, toast the sesame seeds over medium-high heat, shaking the pan occasionally, until the seeds are fragrant and start to crackle and pop, 4 minutes. Add the toasted sesame seeds to the kale mixture. Using your fingers, massage the mixture for 30 to 60 seconds to combine the ingredients and let the warm seeds help release the essential oils in the thyme.

To store: This condiment keeps in a sealed jar in the refrigerator for 10 days.

CRISPED KALE, COLLARD GREENS, or BROCCOLI LEAF

MAKES ABOUT 4 CUPS | GF

Crisp-roasted kale tastes like a cross between nori and potato chips. Collards and broccoli leaves, without kale's bitterness, taste even better. This low-heat method leaves more of the nutrients in the greens. Besides eating these as chips, crush these crisp greens over soups, sprinkle on salads, cooked beans, grains, and your morning oatmeal, too. Also add them to popcorn and baked goods like Cayenne Shortbread (p. 30) and Oatmeal Everything Cookies (p. 208).

8 green curly kale leaves or 1 small bunch (8 ounces) Tuscan kale, stems removed, torn into 2-inch pieces (see below for amounts of other greens)

1 tablespoon extra-virgin olive oil

1. Set a rack in the center of the oven. Preheat the oven to 250° F. Line a baking sheet with baking parchment.

2. In a mixing bowl, massage the greens with the oil until they are evenly coated. Spread the greens in one layer on the prepared baking sheet. If edges overlap slightly, it is okay.

3. Bake the kale for 15 minutes. Using tongs, turn and rearrange the pieces. Bake for 15 minutes, and turn the pieces again. Bake until the kale is completely dry and crunchy, up to 15 minutes more. Stored in an airtight tin, crisped greens keep for 5 days.

COOK'S TIP

To double the recipe, use 1 tablespoon oil and spread the greens on 2 baking sheets.

CRISPED COLLARD GREENS

Roll and cut 4 stripped leaves crosswise into ¾-inch strips. Prepare as above. Bake for 15 minutes, turn, and bake 15 to 20 minutes.

BROCCOLI LEAF

Tear 7 leaves into 2-inch pieces. Prepare as above. Bake for 15 minutes, turn, and bake 15 to 20 minutes.

DILL-PICKLED KALE STEMS

MAKES 1/2 PINT |

Thin slices of this sharp, garlic-punctuated pickle add pungent flavor to dishes. Packed in a canning jar, this makes an attractive gift. Use only pieces of stems no more than ¼-inch thick. Anything thicker is too woody and tough.

Green curly kale stem sections ¼ inch thick, cut into 2- to 3-inch lengths

½ cup apple cider vinegar

1 or 2 garlic cloves, halved lengthwise

1 teaspoon sugar

½ teaspoon kosher salt, optional

2 dill heads, fresh or dried, or ¼ teaspoon dill seed, or 2 sprigs fresh dill

1. Pack the kale stems into a ½-pint canning jar to check how many will fit, leaving room to add the garlic and dill. Use the tip of a small knife to mark the stems ½-inch below the rim of the jar.

2. Place the jar and 2-piece canning lid in a pot of boiling water, covering them to a depth of 2 inches, and boil for 10 minutes. Or, run the jar through the dishwasher just before you use it. Leave it there until you fill it.

3. Meanwhile, in a medium saucepan, cook the kale stems in boiling water for 3 minutes. Drain in a colander and run cold water over them until cooled, 1 minute. Drain the stems.

4. In a small saucepan, boil the vinegar, garlic, sugar, and salt (if using), and ½ cup water. Pack the dill into the hot jar. Add the kale stems and the garlic from the hot pickling mixture. Pour in the hot liquid, leaving ¼ inch of space at the top of the jar. Cover the jar and let sit until it is room temperature.

5. Tighten the cap as much as possible. Refrigerate the pickled stems for at least 3 days before using. The longer they sit, the more pungent they will be.

To store: Keep tightly covered in the refrigerator for up to 3 months.

USE THIN SLICES

In potato, egg, tuna, and pasta salads
   On green salads, cottage cheese, or steamed vegetables
   In dips and salsa

COOK'S TIPS

Minerals in sea and table salt can discolor the pickles.
   Stems from other kinds of kale are too tough to pickle.

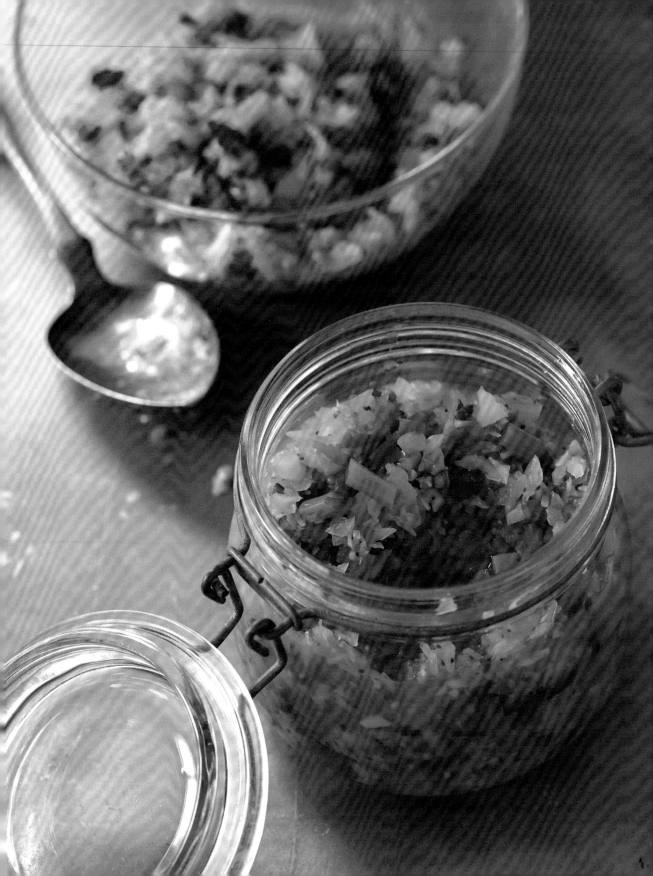

IMPATIENT PICCALILLI

MAKES ABOUT 7 CUPS |

Tomatillos work beautifully in this relish and using them in place of green tomatoes makes this a year-round recipe. A food processor makes quick work of chopping all the vegetables. I call this an "impatient" pickle because you can eat it after 3 days, although it is even better if you age it for the customary 3 weeks. This relish keeps in the refrigerator without canning, but I recommend processing it in a hot water bath if you want to give it as a gift. (For canning directions, see www.freshpreserving.com.)

1 pound green cabbage, cut into 1½-inch chunks

1 pound green tomatoes, or tomatillos, cut into 4 to 8 pieces

1 small green bell pepper, seeded and diced

1 small red bell pepper, seeded and diced

½ pound onions, cubed

1 cup kale stems, stripped clean and cut into ¼-inch pieces

1 cup organic cane sugar or white sugar

1 tablespoon celery seed

1 tablespoon yellow mustard seed

1 to 2 teaspoons ground turmeric

1 dried red hot pepper

1 tablespoon kosher salt

2 cups white vinegar

1. In a food processor, chop the cabbage by pulsing 15 to 20 times, until it resembles confetti. Transfer the cabbage to a large bowl. Chop the tomatoes or tomatillos, green and red peppers, and the onions, one at a time, adding each one to the bowl. Add the kale stems and mix to combine all the vegetables.

2. In a 4-quart stainless steel or other non-reactive saucepan, combine the sugar, celery and mustard seeds, turmeric, hot pepper, salt, and vinegar. Heat the mixture on medium-high heat, stirring just until the sugar dissolves. Add all the chopped vegetables. Increase the heat to bring the relish to a boil as quickly as possible. Reduce the heat so it boils gently, and cook for 15 minutes, stirring a few times, until the relish is crisp-tender. Do not be concerned—the liquid will increase as the relish cooks, until the vegetables are swimming in it. If you like softer relish, cook for 20 minutes.

3. While the piccalilli cooks, immerse 7 half-pint jars and their 2-piece canning lids in a pot of boiling water and boil for 10 minutes, keeping the jars submerged by at least 1 inch of water the entire time. Or run the jars and lids through the dishwasher just before you use them. Leave them there until you fill the jars.

4. Immediately ladle the hot relish into the sterilized jars, seal, and label. Let the jars sit until the piccalilli is completely cooled. If you are not processing it in a hot water bath, keep refrigerated, even before opening.

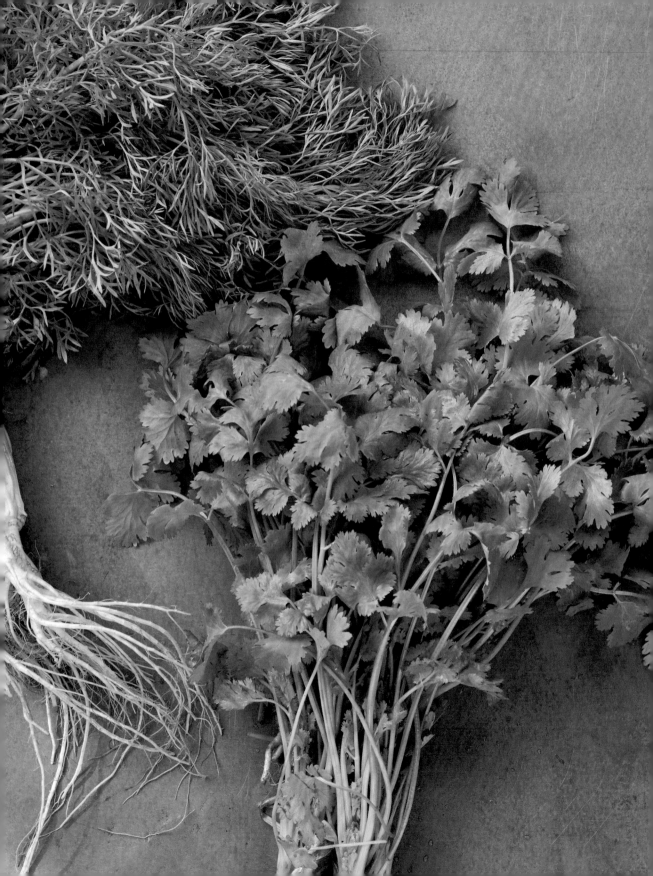

8.
SMALL MEALS and SNACKS

EATING GREENS WITH DINNER IS EASY BUT FITTING THEM into lunch, breakfast, and snacks in significant amounts takes some planning. Here are ways to get your Power Greens during the day without relying solely on salads, soups, and spinach-topped pizza, or by adding a handful of kale to a smoothie.

Greens go well with eggs, scrambled with chopped Short Cooked greens or as lavish amounts of chopped parsley and cilantro in Zucchini, Onion, and Fresh Herb Frittata (p. 191). You can heap a pile of arugula on generous Bacon, Arugula, and Tomato on Focaccia (p. 185) for lunch or breakfast. There are also days when a Cheddar cheese scone including spinach or an open-face sandwich of avocado and watercress is good.

Adding watercress enhances both the flavor and nutrients in the Smoked Salmon, Goat Cheese, and Watercress Wrap (p. 190). Black Bean and Broccoli Leaf Burgers (p. 196) are perhaps the ultimate super-charged veggie burger. Spinach and Corn Pancakes with Lime Drizzle (p. 199) refashions flapjacks as a savory brunch or light dinner dish with a sweet and tart twist. For a comfort-food dinner, have a baked potato stuffed with broccoli rabe and cheese, saving a second one to reheat for breakfast or lunch. Finally, a stack of roasted winter squash slices with a topknot of gingered greens makes a colorful dish for a late brunch or light dinner.

Liquid greens also help you meet the day's target. Mean Green Smoothie (p. 213) has the kick of kimchi, while Glorious Greens Juice (p. 217) deliciously puts a salad in a glass. Sparkling Parsley-Ginger Lemonade (p. 214) made with Parsley Elixir (p. 214) is refreshing and restorative.

BACON, ARUGULA, and TOMATO on FOCACCIA

SERVES 2 | (30)

Focaccia is an ideal base in this greener, improved variation of the classic BLT. Toasted, the focaccia provides a crisp crust and a soft inside that soaks up the juices from the tomato. Hellmann's mayo is fine but using a premium quality one like Sir Kensington or Green Herb Mayonnaise (p. 28) puts this sandwich over the top.

2 4 x 3½-inch pieces of focaccia, halved horizontally

4 slices preservative-free thick-cut bacon, halved crosswise

3 tablespoons Green Herb Mayonnaise (p. 28) or best-quality prepared mayonnaise

2 large beefsteak tomato slices, ¾-inch thick

1 lightly packed cup baby or wild arugula

1. Preheat the oven to 325°F.

2. Place the pieces of focaccia cut side down directly on the oven rack and toast for 7 to 8 minutes, until the bread is crisp and lightly toasted.

3. Meanwhile, in a skillet over medium heat, cook the bacon until it is browned and crisp, about 10 minutes, turning it frequently so it cooks evenly. Drain the bacon on a paper towel.

4. Spread 1½ tablespoons of the mayonnaise to cover the cut side of each toasted focaccia square. Place a tomato slice on each bottom square. Top with 4 pieces of the bacon. Arrange the arugula on top of the bacon. Close each sandwich. Serve immediately.

GOOD TECHNIQUE

Cooking bacon slowly and turning it often melts out the most fat, making the crispest and most evenly browned bacon. Rotate the strips in the pan as well as flipping them over.

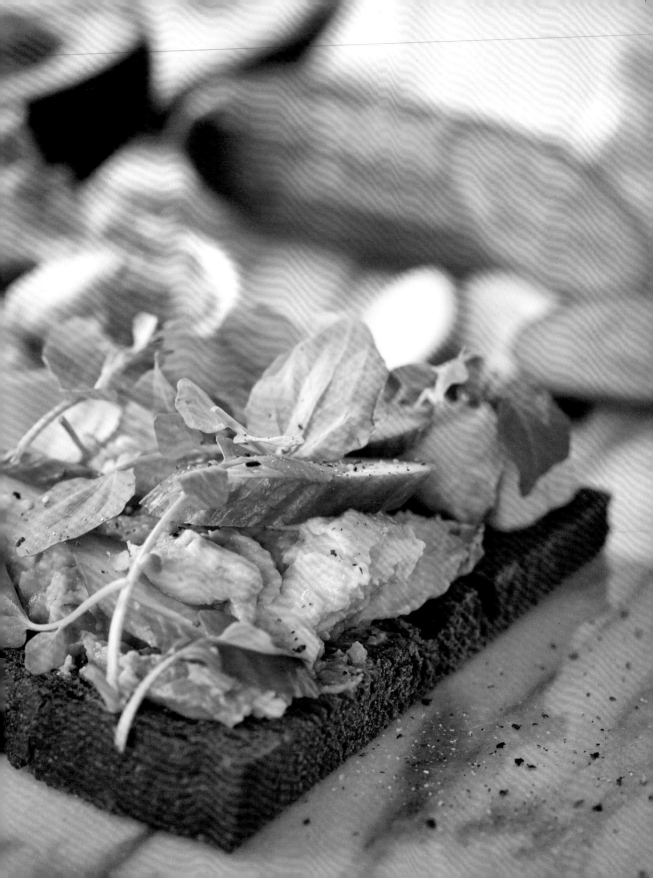

AVOCADO and WATERCRESS TARTINE

SERVES 2 |

Rather than the dainty finger sandwiches served with afternoon tea, this open-face one is generous enough to be a meal. Made on European dark rye bread, it harks back to the days when European peasants relied on sturdy, whole-grain bread and wild watercress they foraged from alongside streams. Lavished with mashed ripe avocado, also called green butter, this sandwich seems more decadent than healthy. Enjoy every bite of its heart-healthy, nutrient-rich fat and the cool cucumber with snappy watercress.

4 square slices European dark rye bread, or 2 long slices halved crosswise

1 Persian cucumber, cut diagonally into thin slices

1 ripe large avocado, pitted, peeled, and cut into 8 wedges

Salt and freshly ground pepper

½ bunch watercress, tough stems removed

1. Lay 2 slices of the bread, or 2 halves of a long slice, on each of two large plates. Arrange 4 of the cucumber slices to cover each bread slice.

2. Place 2 avocado wedges on each piece of bread. Using a fork, mash the avocado. With the back of the fork, spread the avocado to cover the cucumber, and season with salt and pepper. Arrange a generous bunch of watercress sprigs on top of the avocado.

WATERCRESS TACOS
with QUESO FRESCO

SERVES 4 | (GF) (30)

I cannot think of a more colorful breakfast or smarter snack than these warm, soft tacos. Watercress fills them with green energy, and they are a perfect introduction if you are hesitant about eating this snappy green. Pairing it with tomato and cilantro in a corn tortilla makes a delicious combination of Mediterranean and Mexican flavors.

8 corn tortillas

1 tablespoon sesame or canola oil

1 medium onion, chopped (¾ cup)

1 garlic clove, chopped

1 jalapeño or serrano pepper, seeded and chopped

3 large (¾-pound) plum tomatoes, seeded and chopped

Freshly ground pepper

2 cups tender watercress sprigs

16 cilantro sprigs

¼ cup (2 ounces) queso fresco or crumbled feta cheese

1. Preheat the oven to 325°F.

2. Wrap the tortillas in foil and warm them in the oven, 10 minutes.

3. In a medium skillet, heat the oil over medium-high heat. Add the onion and cook, stirring often, until it is translucent, 4 minutes. Add the garlic and hot pepper and cook for 1 minute. Add the tomatoes and cook until they start to break down, 4 minutes. Season with 4 grinds of pepper.

4. To serve, put 2 tortillas on each of four dinner plates. Divide the tomato mixture evenly among the tortillas. Top with one-fourth of the watercress. Add the cilantro sprigs and sprinkle on the cheese. Top each taco with ⅛ of the watercress.

NUTRINOTE

Only organic corn is not genetically engineered, so I suggest using the whole-grain organic tortillas from Food For Life. They also have the best, full corn flavor along with providing 3 grams of fiber. Look for them in the freezer case at natural food stores.

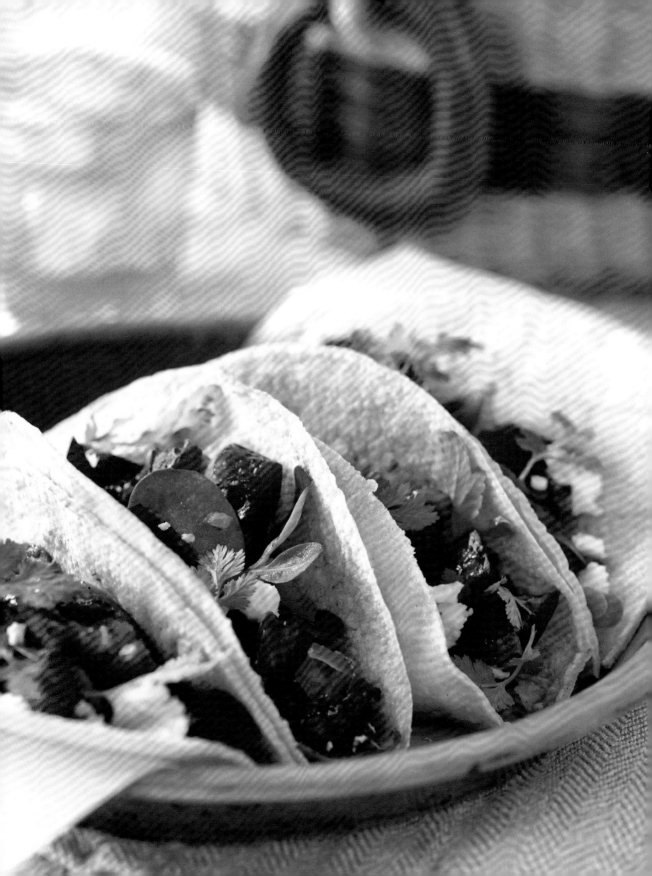

SMOKED SALMON, GOAT CHEESE, and WATERCRESS WRAP

SERVES 4 | (30)

Salmon has so many health benefits that eating it regularly is essential. Since smoked salmon is costly, this quickly assembled wrap helps make the most of it. Including a schmear of creamy cheese plus whole grain in the wrap, it turns lunch at your desk or an impromptu picnic into a luxury moment.

2 whole-wheat or multigrain flatbread wrappers

2½ ounces fresh goat cheese, about a 3-inch piece of a log

Freshly ground pepper

4 ounces sliced smoked wild coho salmon

10 to 12 sprigs watercress, tough stems removed

3-inch piece Persian cucumber, peeled and quartered lengthwise

½ cup grape tomatoes, optional, for garnish

1. Lay a wrapper on your work surface with a narrow end toward you. Spread it with half the goat cheese, leaving a 1-inch border across the top. Add 3 or 4 grinds of pepper. Arrange half the salmon over the cheese, covering about two-thirds of the wrap starting from the bottom.

2. Arrange half the watercress 1 inch above the bottom edge across the salmon. Lay two cucumber spears alongside the watercress. Lifting the bottom edge, roll the flatbread up, pressing with your fingers against the cress and cucumber to make a tight roll. Repeat to make the second wrap.

3. To serve, trim off the ends and cut each wrap diagonally into 2 pieces, and arrange on four plates. Garnish each plate with half the grape tomatoes, if desired.

To store: Serving these wraps freshly made is best, but you can wrap them in plastic wrap and refrigerate for up to 2 hours.

COOK'S TIP

You do not need fancy, hand-sliced salmon for this wrap. The packaged, sliced wild salmon from Costco, Trader Joe's, or the supermarket is just fine.

ZUCCHINI, ONION, and FRESH HERB FRITTATA

SERVES 6 |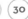

Egyptian cooks make a frittata, which they call an *eggah,* even better by browning the onion and squash, giving an edge to their sweetness. They also add lots of chopped fresh herbs, especially dill and parsley. This frittata tastes good when slightly cooled and even better at room temperature. Try it also sandwiched into a length of buttered, crusty French bread lined with red leaf lettuce.

6 large eggs

3 tablespoons extra-virgin olive oil

1 medium onion, halved and thinly sliced

1 medium (6-ounce) zucchini, thinly sliced

½ teaspoon ground cumin

¼ teaspoon ground turmeric

½ teaspoon salt

Freshly ground pepper

½ cup coarsely chopped flat-leaf parsley

¼ cup snipped fresh dill

1. In a medium bowl, whisk the eggs.

2. In a medium skillet that can go under the broiler, heat 1 tablespoon of the oil. Add the onion and cook, stirring often, until it is golden and starting to brown, 8 minutes. Add the onion to the eggs.

3. Add 2 teaspoons oil to the pan. Spread the zucchini in an even layer and cook for 2 minutes. Using tongs to turn the slices as they brown on the bottom, cook until the zucchini is lightly browned on both sides and looks translucent, about 4 minutes. Add the zucchini to the eggs. In a small bowl, mix the cumin and turmeric with 1 teaspoon warm water, then mix the spices into the eggs. Add the salt and 5 or 6 grinds of pepper. Mix in the parsley and dill.

4. Wipe out the pan with a moist paper towel and return it to the heat. Add the remaining 4 teaspoons oil. Pour in the egg mixture and cook over medium heat until the eggs are set around the sides of the frittata. Run a wide spatula around the sides and ease it under the bottom, then continue cooking until the frittata is well set on the bottom but still runny on top in the center, 8 minutes. Slide the frittata pan under the broiler just until the top is set and golden, 1 minute. Cut the frittata into 6 wedges and serve.

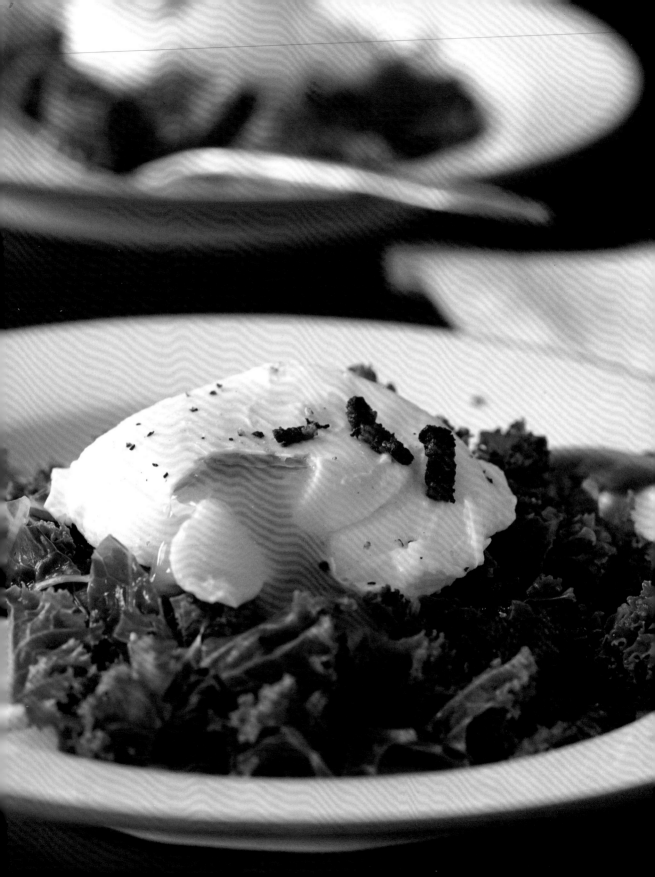

POACHED EGGS in a NEST of BACON-WILTED KALE

SERVES 4 | GF 30

You can fry the egg in this breakfast, lunch, or dinner dish but it is even better poached. For complete bliss, serve with hash brown potatoes made with bacon fat.

2 slices preservative-free bacon, cut into ½-inch pieces

1 small bunch (8 ounces) green kale, stem and center veins removed

½ cup fat-free reduced-sodium chicken broth, or water

1 tablespoon white vinegar

Salt

4 large eggs, cold and as fresh as possible for thicker whites

Freshly ground pepper

1. In a heavy medium skillet, cook the bacon over medium heat until crisp, 8 minutes. Drain the bacon on paper toweling. Pour off the bacon fat, reserving 2 tablespoons in the pan.

2. In a large covered saucepan, boil 8 cups of water. Add the kale, using a wooden spoon to push it into the water until the leaves collapse. Cover and cook for 4 minutes over medium-high heat. Drain the kale in a colander, then run cold water over it while swishing with your hand until the greens feel cool, 30 seconds. Squeeze the kale to remove excess water. Chop the kale finely and pull it apart; there will be about 1 cup.

3. In the pan with the bacon fat, spread the kale in an even layer. Add the broth or water and cook over medium-high heat, stirring occasionally, until the kale is fluffy and dry, about 10 minutes. Season with salt and pepper. Arrange one-fourth of the kale in a ring on each of four plates.

4. To poach the eggs, pour 8 cups water into the skillet used for the kale. Add the vinegar and 1 teaspoon salt. Bring the liquid to a boil, then reduce the heat until the water is barely simmering. Crack each egg into a saucer, then slide it into the hot water. Keep the water at a bare simmer; do not let it boil. After 1 minute, use a spatula to gently loosen the eggs from the bottom of the pan. Cook for 2 to 4 minutes. With a slotted spoon, transfer the eggs to the kale nests. Sprinkle the bacon over and around each egg and serve.

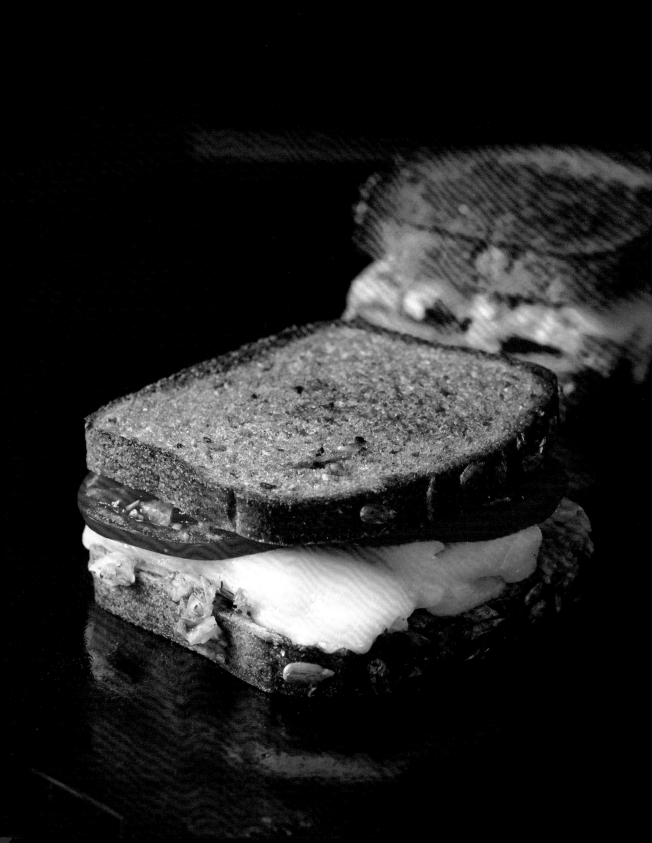

GRILLED CHEESE and TOMATO SANDWICH with KIMCHI

SERVES 1 | (VG) (30)

Kimchi brings the wow to this toasted cheese and tomato sandwich. If you have never had this umami-rich Korean fermented cabbage, it is a perfect introduction.

1½ tablespoons unsalted butter, softened

2 slices whole-grain sandwich bread

½ cup kimchi, well-drained and finely chopped

2 ounces Monterey Jack cheese, thinly sliced

2 thin tomato slices

1. Heat a medium cast-iron skillet or stovetop griddle over medium-high heat.

2. Butter the bread slices on one side. Place the bread, buttered side down, in the hot pan. Arrange the kimchi to cover one slice of the bread. Cover the kimchi with the cheese slices. Place the tomato slices on top of the cheese. Close the sandwich with the second slice of bread, placing it buttered side up.

3. Using a wide spatula, press the sandwich, then carefully turn it. Press again, and cook until the cheese is soft and the bottom of the sandwich is well-browned, 1 to 2 minutes. Turn the sandwich again and cook until the cheese is melted and the sandwich is well-browned on the second side, about 2 minutes. Transfer the sandwich to a plate, cut it diagonally in half, and serve.

NUTRINOTE

The liquid from kimchi is rich in probiotics. Save it to add to tomato juice or mix into a bowl of vegetable soup.

BLACK BEAN and BROCCOLI LEAF BURGERS

SERVES 8 |

Veggie burgers made from scratch are often held together by an abundance of breadcrumbs that make them as hard and dry as a hockey puck. Or they are moist but they fall apart. To make an ideal veggie burger that holds together, I have discovered that very soft-cooked rice is the magic ingredient. Making these veggie burgers takes time but they are so crusty and satisfying that they are worth it. In addition to being delicious, they are a protein powerhouse, and rich in fiber, too.

1 cup frozen brown rice

½ cup frozen shelled edamame

⅓ cup frozen corn kernels

4 large or 6 medium fresh broccoli leaves, stems and center veins removed

3 tablespoons canola oil

1 medium red onion, finely chopped

1 large garlic clove, finely chopped

1 15½-ounce can black beans, drained

¼ cup ground almonds

1 teaspoon ground paprika

¼ to ½ teaspoon ancho chile powder, or ⅛ teaspoon cayenne pepper

½ cup (2 ounces) shredded low-fat sharp Cheddar cheese

Salt and freshly ground pepper

8 5-inch whole-wheat pita breads

4 cups finely shredded romaine lettuce

8 tomato slices

8 red onion slices

Ketchup, optional

1. In a small saucepan, cook the rice with ¼ cup water, covered, until it is very soft, about 8 minutes. Place the rice in the bowl of a food processor.

2. In another small saucepan, cook the edamame and corn with ⅓ cup water, covered, over medium-high heat until they are soft, 8 minutes. Drain the vegetables and set aside.

3. Meanwhile, in a covered large saucepan, boil 6 cups of water over high heat. Add the broccoli leaves, using a wooden spoon to push them into the water. Cover, reduce the heat to medium-high, and cook for 4 minutes. Drain the leaves in a colander, then run cold water over them while swishing with your hand until they feel cool, 30 seconds. Gather the leaves and squeeze them to remove excess water. Chop the broccoli leaves finely and pull them apart; there will be about 1 cup.

4. In a large skillet, heat 1 tablespoon of the oil over medium-high heat. Cook the onion until translucent, 4 minutes. Add the garlic and cook until the onion is soft, 4 minutes. Add the onion and garlic to the food processor with the rice. Wipe out the pan and set it aside.

5. Add the beans to the food processor and pulse until the mixture is coarsely chopped. Add the edamame and corn, almonds, paprika, and chile powder and pulse just to blend,

6 pulses. Add the cheese and pulse to blend, 4 pulses. Transfer the burger mixture to a medium bowl. Season the mixture with salt and pepper.

6. Lightly moisten your hands and shape the burger mixture into 8 patties. At this point, the burgers can be covered with plastic wrap and refrigerated for up to 24 hours.

7. To cook the burgers, heat the remaining 2 tablespoons of oil in the skillet over medium-high heat. Place the burgers ½ inch apart in the pan and cook until they are crusty on the bottom, 4 minutes. Using a wide spatula, turn the burgers and brown well on the second side, 3 to 4 minutes.

8. To serve, pull open the pita breads and line each one with ½ cup of the lettuce. Add a burger, a tomato slice, and an onion slice. If desired, add ketchup.

COOK'S TIP

Instead of frozen rice, you can cook 3 tablespoons of short-grain brown rice in 1¼ cups water until it is very soft, 45 minutes. This can be done up to 8 hours ahead.

TURKEY SLIDERS

SERVES 6 |

I call these juicy burgers "White Castle meets La Dolce Vita." Onions give them flavor reminiscent of the little patties from White Castle. The topping is inspired by extravagantly overloaded burgers that I ate at a *caffé* on the *Via Condotti* in Rome, served on a soft egg bun and layered with ketchup, mayonnaise, and mustard. Using bread in the burger mixture, like when making a meatloaf, keeps these burgers light and juicy while also helping you eat more whole grain. On-the-vine tomatoes produce slices that are just the right size.

½ package (5 ounces) defrosted frozen chopped spinach

1 small onion, coarsely grated

2 slices whole-wheat sandwich bread, crusts removed, cut into ½-inch pieces

1 teaspoon salt

Freshly ground pepper

1 pound 90 to 94% lean ground turkey

½ cup (2 ounces) shredded sharp Cheddar cheese

2 teaspoons extra-virgin olive oil

12 mini burger buns, preferably whole-wheat, toasted

Romaine lettuce, torn into 3-inch pieces

12 small tomato slices, such as from on-the-vine tomatoes

Ketchup, brown mustard, and mayonnaise, optional

1. Squeeze the moisture from the spinach, chop it finely, then fluff it with your fingers. Place the spinach in a mixing bowl. Gently squeeze most of the moisture from the onion and add it to the bowl. Add the bread, the salt, and 4 or 5 grinds of pepper, and mix to combine with the vegetables. Add the turkey, and using a fork, mix to combine it with the other slider ingredients. Mix in the cheese. Using a ¼-cup measure, scoop up and form the mixture into 12 loosely knit patties. At this point, the patties can be covered with plastic wrap, arranged in one layer on a plate, and refrigerated for up to 4 hours.

2. In large skillet, heat the oil over medium-high heat. Arrange the sliders in the pan and cook until browned on the bottom, about 5 minutes. Turn and cook until the patties are no longer pink in the center, about 4 minutes. Cook the sliders in two batches, if necessary.

3. To serve, set a slider on the bottom half of each bun. Top with a piece of lettuce and a tomato slice. Add ketchup, mustard, and mayonnaise, according to your taste.

SPINACH and CORN PANCAKES with LIME DRIZZLE

SERVES 4 | (VG) (30)

For brunch or a light dinner, enjoy these savory pancakes topped with a tart-sweet syrup. Folding in a whipped egg white makes these vegetable-studded flapjacks exceptionally light and fluffy.

¾ cup unbleached all-purpose flour

2 tablespoons baking powder

1 large egg, plus 1 white

⅔ cup reduced-fat (2%) milk

½ teaspoon salt

5 tablespoons unsalted butter, melted

⅓ cup frozen yellow corn kernels, defrosted

8 ounces frozen chopped spinach, defrosted and squeezed dry

3 tablespoons chopped scallions, green part only

Canola oil or cooking spray

2 tablespoons dark agave syrup

1 tablespoon fresh lime juice

1. In a medium bowl, whisk together the flour and baking powder. In a 2-cup measuring cup, add the whole egg to the milk and beat with a fork to combine them. Mix in the salt and 4 tablespoons of the melted butter. Pour the liquid ingredients into the dry and whisk just until combined; a few lumps are better than overmixing.

2. Blot the corn dry on a paper towel and add it to the batter. Add the spinach and scallions and whisk gently to distribute the vegetables in the batter.

3. In a clean, dry bowl use a clean whisk to whip the egg white into soft peaks. Gently fold the beaten white into the batter.

4. Heat a large skillet or griddle over medium-high heat. Lightly coat the pan with oil. Using a ¼-cup measure, drop 3 tablespoons of the batter into the pan for each pancake, spacing the pancakes 3 inches apart to allow space for spreading. When the undersides of the pancakes are browned and bubbles appear on the top, use a wide spatula to flip the pancakes. Cook until browned on the bottom, 1 to 5 minutes. If desired, hold the pancakes in a preheated 200°F oven while cooking the rest of the batch.

5. For the syrup, in a small bowl, combine the agave, lime juice, and remaining 1 tablespoon melted butter. Divide the pancakes among four plates. Drizzle one-fourth of the syrup over each serving.

SPINACH and CHEDDAR SCONES

MAKES 9 SCONES |

Buttery and rich with cheese, these golden scones flecked with spinach are decadent with a nice, strong cup of tea. Or split one open like an English muffin and top each half with a slice of roasted turkey as a change from the usual sandwich.

8 tablespoons (1 stick) unsalted butter

2½ cups unbleached, all-purpose flour

2½ teaspoons baking powder

1 teaspoon sugar

½ teaspoon salt

¾ cup reduced-fat (2%) milk

½ cup shredded sharp Cheddar, full fat or light

½ cup finely chopped raw baby spinach

2 tablespoons snipped chives

1. Place a rack in the center of the oven. Preheat the oven to 400°F. Lightly coat a baking sheet with cooking spray and set aside.

2. Cut the butter into small cubes and place in the freezer to chill while you measure the other ingredients.

3. In a large bowl, whisk together the flour, baking powder, sugar, and salt. Add the chilled butter and, using a pastry blender, your fingertips, or two knives, work it into the dry ingredients until the combination resembles coarse meal, about 2 minutes, rotating and tilting the bowl as you work.

4. Add the milk, cheese, spinach, and chives and mix gently with a fork, then your fingers, to make a clumpy dough, reaching down to incorporate the dry ingredients from the bottom of the bowl. Set aside for 5 minutes to let the dough become softer.

5. Turn out the dough onto a lightly floured surface and use your fingers to work in any loose bits while handling it as little as possible. Press the dough into an 8-inch square that is ¾-inch thick. With a sharp knife, cut the dough into 9 squares.

6. Transfer the scones to the prepared baking sheet. Bake for 25 minutes, until the scones are golden brown. Cool the scones on a wire rack. Serve warm or at room temperature.

POWER OATMEAL

SERVES 2 | (V) (30)

Nutty and chewy, this steel-cut oatmeal makes a sturdy breakfast rich in slow-burning complex carbs. At a B&B serving macrobiotic food, I discovered that nori sprinkled on oatmeal along with raisins and brown sugar is delicious. Crisped kale tastes even better. Ready in 15 minutes, this also makes a comforting dinner.

¼ teaspoon salt

½ cup quick-cooking steel-cut oats

1 tablespoon dried currants

1 tablespoon golden raisins

1 tablespoon chopped walnuts

2 teaspoons chia seeds

2 teaspoons coconut sugar or packed brown sugar

⅓ cup Crisped Kale (p. 178)

2 teaspoons chilled unsalted sweet butter, cut into very thin slices, optional

1. In a small saucepan, boil 2½ cups water. Add the salt. Mix in the oatmeal. Simmer the oatmeal, uncovered, for 10 minutes, stirring it 3 or 4 times. Cover and set aside for 3 minutes.

2. Meanwhile, in a small bowl, combine the currants, raisins, walnuts, chia seeds, and sugar. Holding the kale, a few leaves at a time, over the bowl, crush it in your fist, then mix to combine with the rest of the topping.

3. Divide the oatmeal between 2 bowls. Top it with the butter, if using. Sprinkle the topping over the oatmeal. Serve immediately.

NUTRINOTE

This whole-grain oatmeal provides more than 4 grams of protein and more than 6 grams of fiber.

ROASTED WINTER SQUASH with GINGER-BRAISED GREENS

SERVES 4 | GF

At a James Beard Foundation Food Conference about sustainability and promoting local agriculture, the chef served a dish he called Winter Squash Napoleon that was stacked slices of roasted squash topped with a tangle of dark greens. While duplicating his dish requires many steps, they are all simple and the result is wicked good. Surround the squash with sautéed cremini mushrooms to make it a meatless main course. Or, for meat eaters, add a lamb chop or beef filet alongside.

1 butternut squash with long neck

1 large Jewel or Garnet yam

1 large yellow summer squash

1 medium Delicata squash or butternut squash

Olive oil or cooking spray

Salt and freshly ground pepper

1 tablespoon extra-virgin olive oil

1 tablespoon finely chopped onion

1 small garlic clove, finely chopped

½ teaspoon grated fresh ginger

3 or 4 chard leaves, stems and center veins removed, coarsely chopped

½ of a 10-ounce bag spinach, stemmed and coarsely chopped

1 chunk Parmigiano-Reggiano cheese, for shaving, optional

1. Preheat the oven to 375°F. Line a baking sheet with baking parchment.

2. Cut 8 slices, each ¾-inch thick, from the neck of the butternut squash, and 4 slices each from the widest part of the yam, the belly of the yellow squash, and from the middle of the Delicata squash. If you do not have Delicata squash, cut 12 slices of butternut squash.

3. Using a swivel-bladed vegetable peeler, peel the yam and butternut squash slices. If some are larger than others, keep peeling around them to make them closer in size. Use a teaspoon to scoop the seeds from the Delicata slices, making rings.

4. Brush the parchment paper with oil or coat it with cooking spray. Arrange the sliced vegetables on the prepared pan, leaving 1 inch between slices. Brush the slices generously with oil or coat them with cooking spray, turn, and coat the second side. Season the slices lightly with salt and freshly ground pepper. Roast the squash for 20 to 25 minutes, until the vegetables are just tender. Set the roasted squash aside.

5. While the squash roasts, heat the 1 tablespoon of oil in a medium skillet over medium-high heat. Add the onion, garlic, and ginger and cook, stirring often, until fragrant, 1 minute. Add the chard and cook, stirring, until it collapses.

continued on page 204

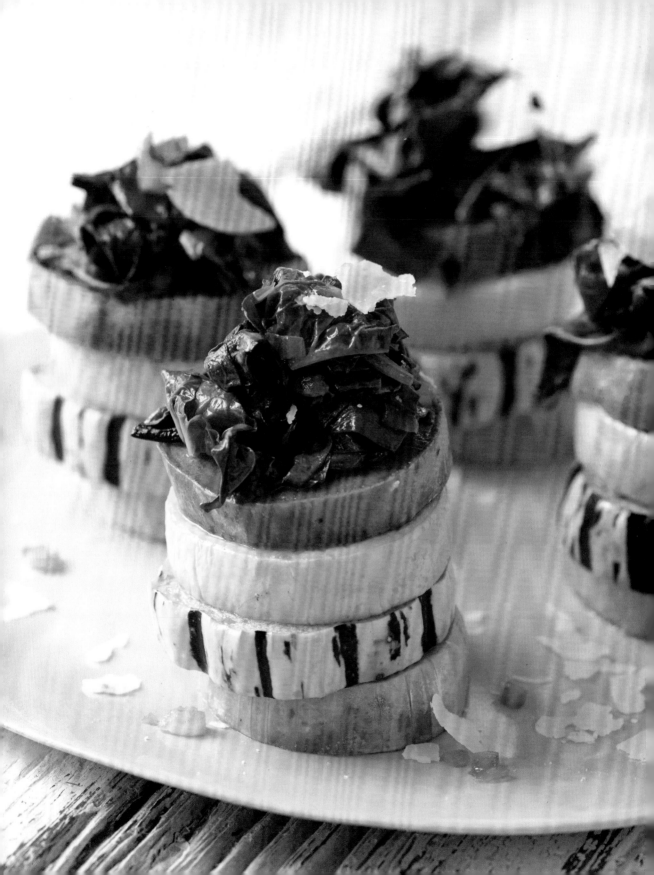

Mix in the spinach. Sprinkle on 1 tablespoon water, and cook until the greens are just tender, about 8 minutes, stirring frequently. Set the cooked greens aside until cool enough to handle. Squeeze most of the moisture from the greens. There should be about 1 cup.

6. To serve, place a slice of butternut squash on a plate. Top it with a slice of Delicata squash (or butternut, if you are not using Delicata), yellow squash, then yam. Add a mound of the greens, using about one-fourth. Repeat, making three more stacks. Using the vegetable peeler, shave four fat curls from the chunk of cheese, and set one on top of each stack. Serve immediately.

COOK'S TIPS

Keep the squash rounds close in size, or your stack will be more of a leaning tower.

Roast the extra squash on a separate pan at the same time as the rounds for this dish. It will keep covered in the refrigerator for 4 days.

TWICE-BAKED POTATO with BROCCOLI RABE

SERVES 4 |

Comfort food with an Italian accent, this crisped potato overloaded with greens and cheese is a meal on its own. Serve it for breakast as well as at lunch or for dinner. Chard, broccoli leaf, or arugula can replace the broccoli rabe, if you wish.

2 large russet potatoes, 10 to 12 ounces each

2 tablespoons extra-virgin olive oil, plus ½ teaspoon

½ bunch (12 ounces) broccoli rabe, tough stems removed

2 garlic cloves, chopped

½ cup (2 ounces) shredded Asiago cheese

Salt and freshly ground pepper

1. Place a rack in the center of the oven. Preheat the oven to 400°F.

2. Coat the potatoes with ½ teaspoon of the oil, or use cooking spray. With the tip of a small knife, pierce the potatoes in four places. Bake the potatoes until the skin is crisp and a knife slips very easily through the inside, 60 to 70 minutes.

3. While the potatoes bake, boil 4 cups of water in a covered, large saucepan. Add the broccoli rabe, using a wooden spoon to push it into the water until the leaves collapse. Cover and cook for 4 minutes over medium-high heat. Drain the broccoli rabe in a colander. Set the bowl under cold running water and swish with your hand until cooled, 30 seconds. A handful at a time, press to extract the excess water from the broccoli rabe. Finely chop the broccoli rabe, then pull it apart; there will be about 1 cup. Give the broccoli rabe a final squeeze.

4. Shortly before the potatoes are done, in a medium skillet, heat the 2 tablespoons oil over medium-high heat. Add the garlic and cook, stirring often, until it colors lightly, 5 minutes. Transfer the garlic to a paper towel and set aside. Add the broccoli rabe to the pan and cook, stirring often, for 2 minutes. Scoop the contents of the pan into a mixing bowl.

5. When the potatoes are done, halve them lengthwise. Scoop their flesh into the bowl with the broccoli rabe,

continued on next page

leaving ¼ inch in the shells. Reduce the oven temperature to 350°F.

6. Add the garlic and half of the cheese to the bowl, and with a fork, mash until the potatoes and broccoli rabe are well-combined. Mash until the mixture is fluffy, 2 minutes. Season the filling with salt and pepper. Spoon all of the filling into the potato shells, smoothing the tops with the back of the spoon.

7. Place the stuffed potatoes on a baking sheet. Sprinkle on the remaining cheese. Bake until the cheese melts, 8 minutes. Serve the potatoes immediately.

To store: Leftover stuffed potatoes can be wrapped in foil and refrigerated for up to 2 days. Add some more shredded cheese, reseal the foil, and reheat the cold potatoes in a 350°F oven for 25 minutes.

FIVE-SPICE BROCCOLI LEAF CHIPS

MAKES 4 CUPS |

Chinese five-spice powder gives these crisp chips flavor that won't let you stop eating them. Using a low-heat oven to bake the chips helps to preserve the fresh taste of the leaves. For a stronger greens flavor, use green curly kale.

6 broccoli leaves (about 8 ounces), stems and center veins removed

1 tablespoon avocado oil or extra-virgin olive oil

¼ teaspoon Chinese five-spice powder

¼ teaspoon grated fresh ginger, optional

Fine sea salt, optional

1. Preheat the oven to 250°F. Line a baking sheet with baking parchment.

2. Tear the broccoli leaves into 2-inch pieces. In a small bowl, combine the oil, five-spice powder, and ginger. Pour the oil over the greens and massage them gently until all the leaves are evenly coated with the flavored oil. Spread the broccoli leaves in an even layer on the prepared baking sheet. It is fine if the pieces overlap slightly. As they dehydrate, they will shrink and get fully exposed to the heat.

3. Bake the broccoli leaves for 15 minutes. Using tongs, turn and rearrange them in an even layer. Bake for 15 to 20 minutes, or until all the pieces are thoroughly dried and crunchy. Transfer the broccoli leaf chips to a bowl. Sprinkle with salt to taste, if desired.

To store: Stored in an airtight tin, these chips keep for 5 days.

OATMEAL EVERYTHING COOKIES

MAKES 12 4-INCH COOKIES |

These big, fat cookies with their crisp edges and chewy centers are inspired by the sublime Compost Cookie from Momofuku Milk Bar in New York City. To the oats, chocolate chunks, potato chips, and ground coffee in the original, I add whole-wheat flour and toss in raisins, peanuts, and Crisped Collard Greens (p. 178). If the crushed greens seem fanciful, their toasted flavor is part of what makes people call these the best cookies ever.

⅓ cup whole-wheat pastry flour

¼ cup unbleached white flour, plus 1 tablespoon

½ teaspoon salt

¼ teaspoon baking powder

¼ teaspoon baking soda

1 teaspoon ground coffee, regular or decaf (not instant)

½ cup organic or white granulated sugar

½ cup lightly packed brown sugar

8 tablespoons (1 stick) unsalted butter, at room temperature

1 large egg

½ teaspoon vanilla extract

½ cup dark chocolate chips

½ cup quick-cooking oats

½ cup coarsely chopped salted peanuts

½ cup roughly crushed potato chips

½ cup raisins

1 cup Crisped Collard Greens or Crisped Kale, lightly crushed (see p. 178)

1. In a small bowl, whisk together the whole-wheat and white flours, salt, baking powder, baking soda, and coffee. Set aside.

2. In the bowl of a stand mixer fitted with the paddle attachment, beat the sugars and butter together on medium-high for 3 minutes. Add the egg and vanilla, and beat for 7 minutes.

3. Add the dry ingredients, and using slow speed, blend just until they combine with the butter mixture. Add the chocolate chips, oats, peanuts, potato chips, and raisins. Add the crisped greens, crushing them a bit more. Using a flexible spatula, mix to combine the greens with the cookie dough.

4. Line 2 cookie sheets with baking parchment. Using a ¼-cup measure, form the dough into 12 balls about the size of a fresh plum and drop them onto the prepared baking sheets, spacing them 4 inches apart. With your fingers, slightly flatten each ball of dough, making 2½ x 1-inch disks. Cover with plastic wrap and refrigerate for 2 to 24 hours.

5. Set a rack in the center of the oven. Preheat the oven to 375°F.

6. Bake the cookies, one sheet at a time, for 16 minutes, or until they are lightly browned around the edges but slightly soft in the centers. Cool the cookies entirely on the baking sheet. Repeat to bake the second sheet of cookies. Stored in an airtight tin, Oatmeal Everything Cookies keep for 5 days. These cookies ship well.

The power of a stand mixer is necessary to give this cookie dough the right texture. Beating it for the specified times and refrigerating the unbaked cookies are also essential. Baking the cookies one sheet at a time ensures their seductive combination of crisp edges and chewy centers.

Be sure to use whole-wheat pastry flour. Natural food stores and some supermarkets carry it, either from Arrowhead Mills or Bob's Red Mill.

NUTRINOTE

These are not health food, but generous amounts of protein, fiber, and fat help to slow down the sugar hit in these cookies.

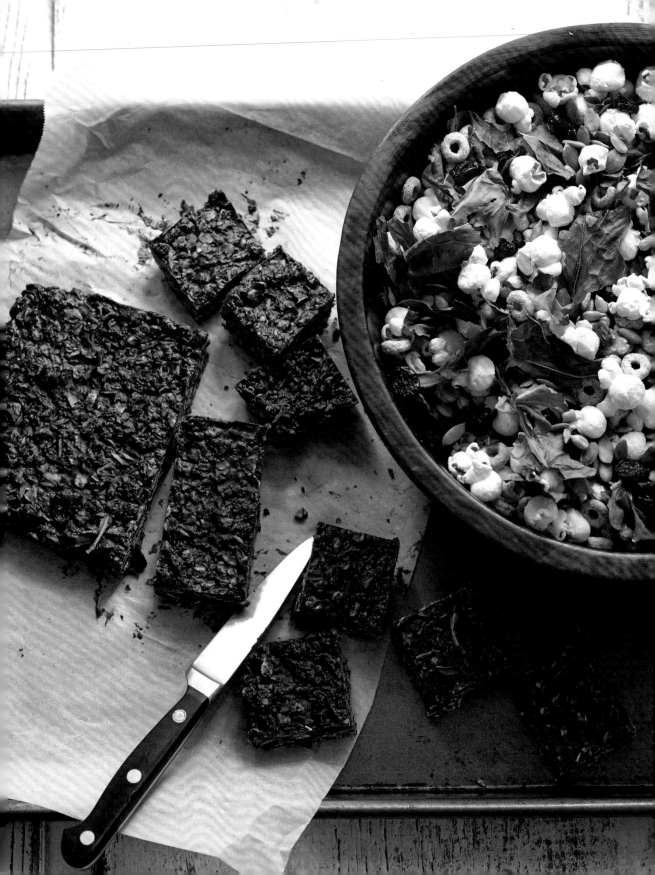

CHOCOLATE FUDGE ENERGY SQUARES

MAKES 16 PIECES |

How can a snack this sinful also be healthy? Easily, when it is loaded with protein from nuts, fiber, and Crisped Kale (p. 178). Serve these energy bombs directly from the refrigerator to keep them firm.

½ cup smooth almond butter

2 tablespoons honey, preferably wildflower

2 tablespoons raw coconut oil

3 to 3½ ounces dark (70%) chocolate, broken up

1 cup old-fashioned rolled oats

¼ cup reduced-fat unsweetened shredded coconut

½ cup dried cranberries, cherries, or raisins

¼ teaspoon salt

¼ cup finely crushed Crisped Kale (see Note)

1. Line an 8-inch loaf pan with parchment paper, using an 8 x 18-inch strip that will cover the bottom and the two long sides of the pan with a couple of inches left for overhang.

2. Combine the almond butter, honey, and coconut oil in a medium saucepan and cook over medium heat until they are warm, stirring with a flexible spatula until they are completely blended, 4 to 5 minutes. Remove from the heat and mix in the chocolate until it melts.

3. Dump in the oats, coconut, dried fruit, and salt, mixing until they are evenly combined with the chocolate mixture. Mix in the kale. Spread the mixture in an even layer in the prepared pan.

4. Chill until the mixture sets into a giant chocolate bar, about 2 hours. Lift the bar out of the pan and cut it crosswise into 8 bars. Cut the bars in half crosswise. Store and serve from the refrigerator.

To store: This snack keeps wrapped both in plastic wrap and then foil in the refrigerator for 5 days.

GOOD TECHNIQUE

To finely crush Crisped Kale (p. 178), hold a quarter-cup measure over a wide bowl, place some kale in the cup, and press it with your fingers, breaking the kale into small bits and flakes. Keep adding and crushing the kale until the cup is full. This will take about 1 cup of Crisped Kale leaves. The bowl keeps things neat.

POPCORN TRAIL MIX

SERVES 4 |

Whether you are hiking a trail or lounging on the couch, this energy-sustaining combination of whole grain, dried fruits, and nuts is fun to munch. Or have it for breakfast, which will make you feel healthfully indulgent. Homemade popcorn is crisper but using store-bought is fine. Kids love to help with making this no-cook mix. Even the littlest ones can participate.

2 cups popcorn

1½ cups unsweetened whole-grain oat cereal

3 tablespoons dried blueberries or golden raisins

3 tablespoons dried cranberries

3 tablespoons Thompson raisins

3 tablespoons chopped walnuts

2 tablespoons roasted pumpkin seeds

2 tablespoons roasted sunflower seeds

2 cups Crisped Collard Greens or Crisped Kale (see p. 178)

In a mixing bowl, combine the popcorn, oat cereal, blueberries, cranberries, raisins, walnuts, pumpkin seeds, and sunflower seeds, using your hands to mix them. Holding the crisped greens over the bowl, lightly crush them, then use your hands to gently mix and combine them.

To store: This snack will keep stored in an open bowl for 2 days, or in a jar for up to 5 days.

COOK'S TIP

Triple the recipe for a party-size batch.

GOOD TECHNIQUE

Roast raw pumpkin seeds in a dry skillet over medium-high heat until they puff up, 3 to 4 minutes.

MEAN GREEN SMOOTHIE

SERVES 1 |

Kimchi gives this smoothie probiotic benefits. Have it to jump-start your morning, keep it in the fridge for lunchtime, or enjoy it as a recharging mid-afternoon snack.

½ cup coconut water

4 romaine lettuce leaves

6 cilantro sprigs

6 flat-leaf parsley sprigs

1 celery rib

¼ ripe avocado

¼ cup kimchi

4 coconut water ice cubes, or plain ice cubes

In a super blender, combine the coconut water, lettuce, cilantro, parsley, celery, avocado, and kimchi, and whirl until smooth. Add the ice cubes and whirl until blended in. Serve in a tall glass, or cover and refrigerate for up to 6 hours.

GOOD TECHNIQUE

Freezing cocunt water or other liquid in cubes to use in drinks keeps their flavor vivid. Freeze, then unmold and store in a resealable plastic bag.

PARSLEY-GINGER LEMONADE

SERVES 4 |

On a hot summer's day, chilled Parsley Elixir (below) brightened with lemon and the zing of ginger is totally thirst-quenching and restorative.

1 recipe Parsley Elixir (below), chilled

Juice of 1 lemon

1 teaspoon grated ginger

Sugar, light agave syrup, or Stevia natural sweetener

4 lemon slices, optional, for garnish

1. In a pitcher, combine the Parsley Elixir, lemon juice, and ginger. Sweeten to taste with your preferred sweetener.

2. To serve, fill four large glasses with ice and divide the lemonade among them. Garnish each glass with a lemon slice, if desired.

COOK'S TIP

Use 1 cup of apple juice instead of a refined sweetener.

PARSLEY ELIXIR

MAKES 3 CUPS |

Actresses drink this herbal infusion to reduce water retention before walking the red carpet. Slightly sweet, it is good served cold or hot, straight or blended with fruit juice.

24 flat-leaf parsley sprigs, preferably organic

3 cups filtered or spring water

Honey, optional

1. Place the parsley and water in a medium saucepan and bring to a boil over medium-high heat. Cover, reduce the heat, and simmer for 1 minute. Steep, covered, for 30 minutes. Uncover and cool to room temperature.

2. Remove the parsley, squeezing it over the pot. Sip the remaining liquid reheated or chilled, sweetened with honey, if desired. It will keep for 4 days covered in the refrigerator. Chilling may turn it cloudy but does not affect the taste.

NUTRINOTE

Parsley is rich in vitamin A, making it good for boosting your immune system.

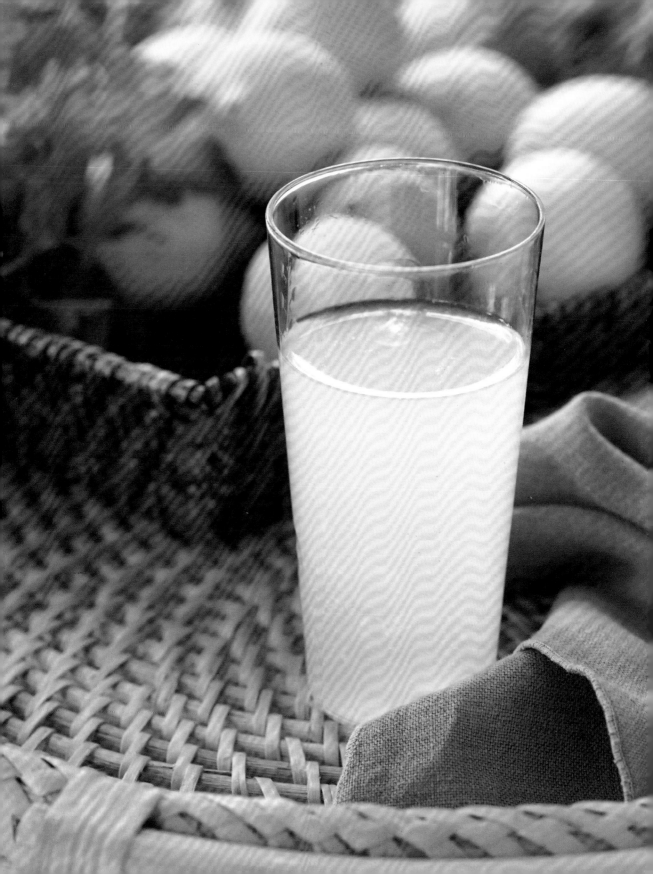

APPLE-PARSLEY TISANE

SERVES 1 |

When your spirits need a lift, wrap your hands around a mug of this warm blend of apple cider and herbal Parsley Elixir and inhale deeply. Even before tasting its natural sweetness, the cozy aroma will cheer you up.

¾ cup Parsley Elixir (p. 214)

⅓ cup fresh apple cider or unfiltered apple juice

Raw cane sugar or coconut sugar

In a small pot, heat the Parsley Elixir, cider, and sweetener over medium-high heat until hot. Serve in a mug.

NUTRINOTE

Vitamins and carotenes in this drink comfort a cold and really can help improve your mood.

GLORIOUS GREENS JUICE

SERVES 1 |

When there is no time to eat a salad, my juicer turns the same ingredients into a fresh drink. Watercress and a Granny Smith apple bring bracing bite and a crisp tang.

7 romaine lettuce leaves

6 inches of cucumber, peeled if not organic

½ bunch watercress

1 Granny Smith apple, cored, preferably organic

Process the lettuce, cucumber, watercress, and apple in a juicer.

To store: This juice keeps covered in the refrigerator for 6 hours.

ASIAN SUPER JUICE

SERVES 1 |

When your immune system needs extra support, give it this liquid boost. Bok choy and apple produce a lot of juice, making this vibrantly green juice budget-friendly.

8 ounces baby bok choy

1 medium Granny Smith or Gala apple

¼ inch fresh ginger

Process the bok choy, apple, and ginger in a juicer.

To store: This juice keeps covered in the refrigerator for 24 hours.

NUTRITIP

According to Jo Robinson, author of *Eating on the Wild Side,* Granny Smith and Gala apples have the most phytonutrients compared to other widely grown commercial varieties

---

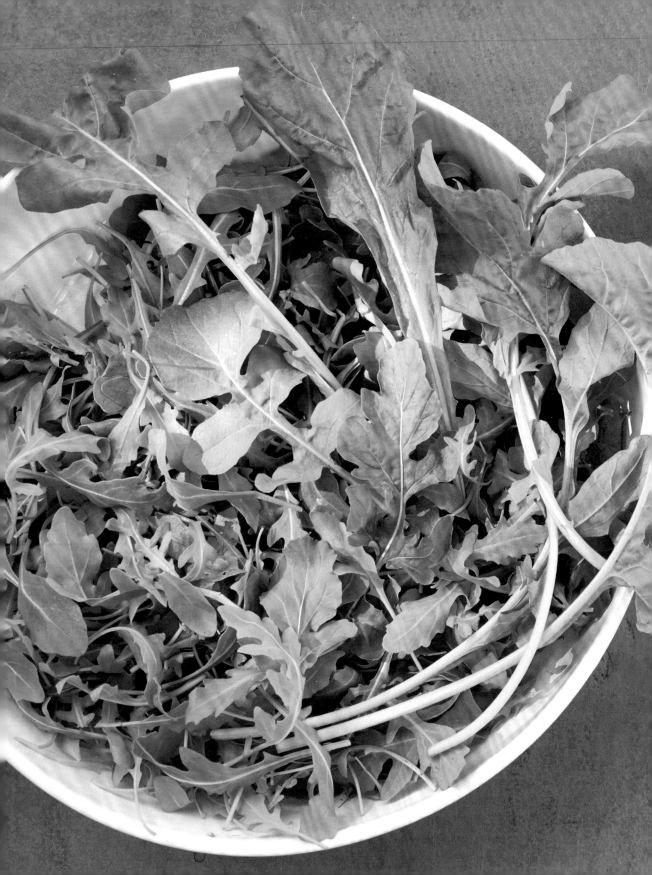

9.

THE BASICS

All About Power Greens, Including How to Buy, Store, and Prep Them

HERE ARE THE PARTICULAR BENEFITS EACH POWER GREEN DELIVERS.

They show why eating all of them is good for you. After you buy them, this is a manual on how to—borrowing the term chefs use—prep your greens, and the best cooking methods for each one. It tells everything you need to use Power Greens in the recipes here and for your own favorite dishes.

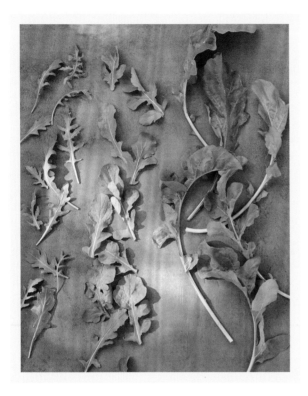

ARUGULA

Arugula has gone from being a gourmet ingredient to an everyday green. It is so popular that packaged salad mixes often include its clean bite. While adding arugula to salads is almost instinctive, I also use it to make a pesto that is good tossed with pasta or steamed vegetables and to bring a green lift to risotto.

What you get: As a brassica, arugula contains important anticancer phytochemicals in addition to good amounts of vitamin A, which helps your immune system; antioxidant vitamin C; folate; magnesium; manganese; and potassium, which helps reduce the risk of high blood pressure. Containing more calcium than any other salad green, plus vitamin K and manganese, arugula helps protect your bones. Adding to its virtues, arugula contains a mere 4 calories per cup.

What to Look For

Pungent, full-grown arugula, milder baby leaves, and fierce wild arugula taste different enough to merit using each of them.

Fully grown arugula looks somewhat like flat-leaf spinach and has a nice bite. Leaves may be ruffled, deeply lobed, or straight-edged and oval, with a hard stem that becomes a tough center vein. It is sold in bunches. When commercially cultivated, this arugula tastes pleasantly nippy. The mature arugula sold at farmer's markets or homegrown turns startlingly hot as the summer goes on, becoming wasabi-sharp. When it bolts, cream-white flowers appear that are heavenly heat bombs.

Baby arugula looks paler, is more tender, and tastes milder. It is sold in plastic boxes or bags at food stores year-round.

Wild arugula, a botanically different plant, has oak leaf–shaped little leaves. It tastes sweet at first, then intensely biting. Look for it at farmer's markets from spring through fall, and, increasingly, in food stores. It may come in a bunch, a plastic box, or loose. A handful has enough zing to stand out.

The phytochemicals that make arugula taste peppery also defend it against predators, so local farmers tend not to spray it. Tiny holes these predators make in the leaves signal that the arugula is unsprayed. They often indicate that it is organically grown, whether mature, baby, or the wild variety.

How to Buy and Store

Look for sprightly, evenly green leaves. Avoid wilted, faded, or yellowing leaves, and bunches with broken stems, torn leaves, or slimy spots, particularly around any bands holding a bunch together. Check bags and boxes for yellowing or rotting leaves, looking especially at the bottom.

Store packaged arugula in its container, adding a paper towel. Unband bunches and store the arugula wrapped in a paper towel in a loosely closed plastic bag, with stem ends facing out in the crisper drawer.

Mature arugula wilts easily, so refrigerate it as quickly as possible and try to use it the day it is bought. Baby arugula sold in a plastic box or bag keeps 3 to 4 days. When sold loose, it may wilt in 2 days. Wild arugula keeps up to 5 days.

Basic Arugula Techniques

WASHING

Wash arugula just before you use it, cleaning only the amount needed. Wash the leaves in a large bowl of cold water. Arugula can be sandy but it bruises easily, so handle leaves gently. Empty and rinse the bowl, then repeat, using 2 or 3 changes of water. Shake the leaves to remove excess water. Rinse arugula even if the package says "triple washed." Spin dry or pat leaves with paper towels.

PREPPING

Mature arugula's tough stem extends as a center vein up through the leaf. Just before using, remove it with the Fold and Tear technique (p. 8). Baby arugula has short stems you can pinch off if you wish. Wild arugula is ready to use.

Chop or tear arugula just before using.

Refrigerate prepped arugula until you are ready to dress and serve salads or add it to a hot dish.

Arugula quickly turns bitter when heated. Instead mix chopped arugula into hot foods to wilt it and release its pungency. Avgolemono Soup with Arugula (p. 48) shows how deliciously this works.

Five Ways to Use Arugula

Top whole-wheat crostini with an onion slice,
baby arugula leaves, and lemon zest

·

Dress corn, tomato, and arugula salad with sherry vinaigrette

·

Drizzle basil oil on a salad of baby arugula,
Granny Smith apple slices, and walnuts

·

Mix baby arugula into mushroom risotto

·

Toss farro with wild arugula and diced beets

ARUGULA RECIPES

FIG AND ARUGULA CROSTINI

HUMMUS WITH ARUGULA AND PARSLEY

AVGOLEMONO SOUP WITH ARUGULA

ARUGULA, ENDIVE, AND AVOCADO SALAD WITH MEYER LEMON VINAIGRETTE

ASPARAGUS, RADISH, AND WATERCRESS SALAD WITH BITTERS VINAIGRETTE

SPICY CHOPPED SALAD

GRILLED EGGPLANT STACKS WITH RED PEPPER, MOZZARELLA, AND ARUGULA PESTO

PAN-SEARED CHICKEN CUTLETS WITH ARUGULA, ORANGE, AND FENNEL

CARROTS WITH WILD ARUGULA PESTO

BACON, ARUGULA, AND TOMATO ON FOCACCIA

BOK CHOY

Choy, which means cabbage in Chinese, refers to an assortment of Asian greens. Bok choy translates as white cabbage. Only bok choy and Shanghai bok choy are featured here because they are the most versatile and the most widely available Asian greens. The distinct flavors of bok choy's mildly pungent stems and its meatier, more intense-tasting leaves are easy to like. Shanghai bok choy tastes even milder and has more tender leaves.

Why it's good: The fleshy, green leaves and crisp, pale stems of these crucifers contain some of the most potent anti-inflammatories found in foods. They include vitamins A and C, and vitamin K, which helps protect cells from damage by free radicals and, along with calcium, makes for strong bones. You also get folate and other B-vitamins. They are good sources of magnesium, which helps muscles relax, potassium, and manganese, along with other minerals. The leaves are rich in lutein and zeaxanthin, carotenoids that protect your eyes.

Phytonutrients in bok choy fight inflammation and stimulate the production of detoxifying enzymes. There are, in addition, substances that help your gut produce immune cells that protect against allergies and inflammatory diseases like arthritis. You get all this for 9 calories per cup.

What to Look For

Bok choy has creamy white, firm stalks 8 to 15 inches tall and deep, mineral-green, crinkled leaves with prominent white veins. A bunch weighs up to 2 pounds.

True baby bok choy is an exact miniature of mature bok choy, with the same white stalks and dark leaves, but in 3- to 6-inch-tall clusters. You rarely see it except in Asian markets. Instead, you often see baby or mature Shanghai bok choy mislabeled as baby bok choy.

Shanghai bok choy comes in clusters with light green, bulbous stalks that narrow to an hourglass shape and pale green, spoon-shaped, flat leaves. Mature Shangai bok choy clusters are 5 to 8 inches tall and weigh 3 to 8 ounces.

How to Buy and Store

Bok choy bunches should feel heavy for their size, with firm stems that are not cracked, bruised, or limp. The leaves should be erect and not yellowed, limp, or full of insect holes. Stems flecked with black dots or dashes are okay.

Shanghai bok choy should have firm, unblemished stems. Its outward curving leaves should be firm and not limp or yellowing.

Organic bok choy, both kinds, is easy to find; using it is recommended.

At home, remove any banding. Store all bok choy wrapped in a paper towel in a loosely closed plastic bag, stem ends toward the opening. If in a plastic box, store it in the box, adding a paper towel once it is opened. Store all bok choy in the produce drawer for up to 5 days.

A large bunch of bok choy, 1 to 1¼ pounds, chopped and stir-fried, serves 4.

For Shanghai bok choy, aka baby bok choy, 1 pound may be 4 to 8 clusters. Braised or stir-fried, whole or chopped, a pound serves four.

Basic Bok Choy Techniques

WASHING

Grit can lodge where the stalks come together at the base of a bunch.

Bok choy: Cut off the bottom inch from the bunch, separating the stalks. Wash bok choy, then shake well and pat dry.

Shanghai bok choy: Trim a thin slice from the base of each cluster. Cut the clusters vertically into halves or quarters and swish in bowl of water, paying careful attention at the bottom, where grit can be lodged. Shake well, then pat dry on paper towels.

PREPPING

For bok choy, separate the leafy tops from the stems. Cut the stems into thin slices to use in salads or into chunky pieces to stir-fry. The tops, cut crosswise into ½-inch ribbons, can be stir-fried or finely shredded and mixed into hot soup or fried rice.

For Shanghai bok choy, leave small clusters whole and halve or quarter larger ones vertically.

COOKING

Bok choy: Stir-fry, sauté, or steam-braise the stems briefly, adding the leaves toward the end. Take care to keep the stems tender-crisp. Serve immediately—cooked bok choy releases a lot of liquid as it stands. Slice the raw stems thinly crosswise and use in salads to add juicy crunch. Add finely shredded leaves to hot dishes, stirring until they wilt.

Shanghai bok choy: Stir-fry, braise, or steam clusters, whole or cut lengthwise. Sometimes I put clusters on an oiled, medium-hot grill until the leaves start to wilt and the stems are marked, then dress the warm, crunchy, chewy clusters with peanut oil.

To add raw to salads, cut clusters of Shanghai bok choy crosswise into ½-inch slices.

Five Ways to Use Bok Choy

Stir-fry bok choy with red bell pepper, red onion,
and ginger black bean sauce

Braise baby bok choy and top it with sautéed shiitake mushrooms

·

Stir-fry bok choy with smoked tofu, scallions, and
peanuts to serve over rice noodles

·

Juice bok choy with ginger, spinach, and green grapes

·

Toss thinly sliced bok choy with black rice, pineapple, radish,
dates, and scallions, and toss with ginger vinaigrette

BOK CHOY RECIPES

HOT AND SOUR SOUP WITH BOK CHOY

BOK CHOY AND CARROT SALAD WITH DOUBLE SESAME DRESSING

CHICKEN SALAD WITH BABY BOK CHOY AND BROCCOLI

RED CHILI TOFU WITH BABY BOK CHOY

GINGER BEEF WITH BOK CHOY

ASIAN SUPER JUICE

BROCCOLI LEAF AND SPIGARIELLO

Broccoli leaves growing on the stalk are as nutrient-rich as the florets they surround, and they taste even better. So does spigariello, an heirloom broccoli that is all leaf and looks more like kale than broccoli. Both these dark greens are sweeter and less bitter than either broccoli or kale while providing even more goodness. If you do not like other Brassicas, these almost black-green leaves will please you.

Broccoli leaves are sold at farmer's markets. Commercially, they are grown by one company, Foxy, and sold as BroccoLeaf in bags at supermarkets and natural food stores.

Spigariello, aka spigarello, is a nonheading broccoli from southern Italy. An Italian-American brought the heirloom vegetable to the U.S. to grow in his home garden. Now, with chefs adoring this substantial yet tender green, farmers in California and in the Northeast are growing it and seed catalogs make it available to home gardeners.

Why it's good: All broccoli leaves contain the phytochemicals that make kale valuable plus ones unique to broccoli, including kaempferol, an antioxidant that helps the body produce detoxifying substances that protect against cancer. They are rich in vitamins A, C, and K, which help blood clot, and folate. A good source of iron, which helps red blood cells carry oxygen, like kale, they are also rich in calcium, potassium, and other minerals.

Pleasing taste, versatility, and all these health benefits make broccoli leaf and spigariello perfect for learning to like cruciferous dark greens.

What to Look For

Broccoli leaves are deep green, with deep notches and rippling edges. Their pale green stem becomes a tough center vein running to the top of the leaf. As BroccoLeaf, they are sold in supermarkets and natural food stores year-round. Loose broccoli leaves sold by farmers growing broccoli appear from fall into the winter months.

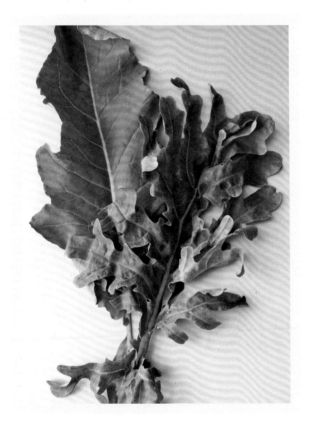

Spigariello is dark bluish green with a hard, round, green stem and a tough center vein that arches so leaves curve backward. Its leaves are spade-shaped, with rippling edges or notched lobes, or curved and twisted like a corkscrew, or skinny and feathered. A bunch of spigariello may include all of these shapes. Spigariello is increasingly available at stores as well as farmer's markets, especially in the eastern United States and on the West Coast, although growing it yourself is the surest way to get it.

How to Buy and Store

Broccoli leaves are sold in bags, bunches, or by the pound. Spigariello comes in bunches or boxed. You want rigid stems supporting fleshy, even-colored dark leaves, possibly with a whitish haze on broccoli leaves. Stems should look fresh-cut at the bottom and not be bruised or cracked. A bunch of spigariello should look animated.

Broccoli leaves collapse in cooking, so a 12-ounce bag makes about 2 cups when Short Cooked. Raw in salads, it serves 4 to 6. Spigariello collapses even more, a 10-ounce bunch making about 1¼ cups when cooked. This makes it a luxury green, but it is so delicious that it's worth the occasional splurge.

For both greens, store the packaged leaves in their bag or box in the crisper drawer of the refrigerator. Remove any banding from bunches. Wrap the leaves loosely in paper towels, slip them into a plastic bag with the stem ends toward the opening, and close the bag loosely. Store broccoli leaves in the coldest part of the refrigerator for up to 4 days. Store spigariello in the crisper drawer for 2 days. Keep them away from apples or other produce that gives off ethylene gas.

Basic Broccoli Leaf Techniques

WASHING

Both kinds of broccoli leaf are usually clean but rinse them in cold running water and shake the leaves dry.

PREPPING

Stripping The stem and center vein of all broccoli leaf are unpleasantly hard. Remove them with the Fold and Tear technique (p. 8)—also best for spigariello's curving leaves—or use the V-Cut (p. 9).

COOKING

Short Cook and Quick Cool both broccoli leaves and spigariello (p. 7). Then braise or add them to soups and stews. Any method good for kale is good for them, as well.

Five Ways to Use Broccoli Leaf and Spigariello

Add braised to a frittata or omelet or when scrambling eggs or tofu

·

Braise and serve with grilled sausages and sweet peppers

·

Make dolmas by wrapping cooked grains in Short Cooked broccoli leaves

·

Simmer and puree broccoli leaves and cauliflower
together for a creamy dairy-free soup

·

Massage shredded broccoli leaves with walnut oil and
add persimmon and pear slices for a winter salad

———

BROCCOLI LEAF RECIPES

BRUSSELS SPROUTS AND BROCCOLI LEAF SLAW

TURKEY SAUSAGE AND PEPPERS WITH SPIGARIELLO

ITALIAN BRAISED GREENS WITH ROASTED GARLIC

SPIGARIELLO WITH PANCETTA

BROCCOLI LEAF, EDAMAME, AND CORN SUCCOTASH

CRISPED KALE, COLLARD GREENS, OR BROCCOLI LEAF

BROCCOLI RABE

Broccoli rabe is also called broccoli raab, rapini, rape, Italian broccoli, or cima di rape. It has lesser-known names as well.

The bitterness of this dark green takes getting used to. For cooks its combination of tender florets, tough leaves, and fibrous stems is unique.

Using the Short Cook–Quick Cool method reduces broccoli rabe's bitterness considerably. Braising it with broth modulates it even further. So does combining broccoli rabe with beans, or grains, as you can see in White Bean and Broccoli Rabe Bruschetta (p. 18) and Seared Polenta with Broccoli Rabe (p. 134).

Broccoli rabe is pricey compared to other greens because sudden weather changes can ruin an entire field in less than 30 minutes, and farmers have to build something into its price to cover likely losses.

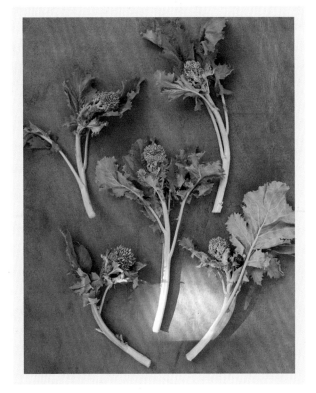

Why it's good: Broccoli rabe is rich in vitamins A, C, K, B-6, which helps the body metabolize carbohydrates, and folate, which is good for your heart. It is a fine source of minerals, including calcium, magnesium, manganese, and potassium. And like all cruciferous vegetables, it contains phytochemicals called isothiocyanates that help the liver neutralize toxins and protect our bodies against cancer and other diseases. You also get 3 grams of protein and 3 grams of fiber in a cup of cooked broccoli rabe.

What to Look For

Select bright green bunches with rigid, mostly thin stems, an abundance of unblemished leaves, and florets with firm, tightly closed buds. Avoid stalks with dry or split ends, yellowed or bruised leaves, and florets with yellow flowers, which mean that the broccoli rabe will be particularly bitter.

How to Buy and Store

All the broccoli rabe sold in supermarkets is grown by the D'Arrigo family and sold under the Andy Boy label. Look for it in bunches and in 5-ounce bags where it is cleaned and ready to cook. A 1¼- to 1½-pound bunch, trimmed and braised, serves 3 to 4. A 5-ounce bag serves 3. At farmer's markets, big bouquets of broccoli rabe abundant with saw-toothed leaves are your best choice.

At home, remove any banding. Store broccoli rabe in a plastic bag with the stem ends toward the opening, adding a paper towel to absorb moisture. Place the loosely closed bag in the coldest part of the refrigerator for no more than 3 days.

Store broccoli rabe away from apples and other fruits giving off ethylene gas.

Basic Broccoli Rabe Techniques

WASHING

Give broccoli rabe a good swish in cold water before or after chopping, then whirl it dry in a salad spinner.

PREPPING

There are three ways to prep broccoli rabe, depending on time and how much you prefer to separate its chewy leaves and tender florets from the fibrous stalks.

The Time-Saving Way Buy bagged, pre-trimmed broccoli rabe. Rinse it, trim any stems that are dry at the bottom, and you're ready to cook.

The Usual Way Pluck off the florets. Holding a handful at a time in one hand on a cutting board, with the other hand, chop off the bottom 1 to 2 inches of stem. Chop the remaining stems and leaves into ¾-inch pieces.

The Perfectionist Way Prepping a bunch of broccoli rabe this way takes 10 minutes to separate the florets, stems, and leaves. It lets you cook each part for just the right amount of time. First, trim off the tough bottom from each stem. Pluck the florets and set aside. Remove the leaves, pile them together, and cut them crosswise into 1-inch strips. Short Cook the stems for 3 to 4 minutes, add the leaves and cook for 2 minutes more, add the florets and cook for 1 minute.

COOKING

When you Short Cook broccoli rabe, the amount of time determines how bitter it tastes. Many recipes have you sauté or steam broccoli rabe just until it collapses, about 5 minutes. The result is bitter and tough. Instead, Short

Cook broccoli rabe and then braise it for 8 minutes (Italian Braised Greens with Roasted Garlic, p. 145). Or braise raw broccoli rabe for 25 minutes when you want stronger flavor.

SHORT COOK–QUICK COOL

In a large saucepan boil 8 cups of water. Add chopped broccoli rabe, pushing it with a wooden spoon until it collapses into the water. Cover and cook over medium-high heat for 4 to 6 minutes, depending on how much bitterness you want to remove. Drain in a colander, then run cold water over the broccoli rabe for 30 seconds. Squeeze the cooled broccoli rabe well; it loves holding on to water.

To finish cooking, steam, sauté, or braise the broccoli rabe.

Steam Sautéing For one bunch of chopped broccoli rabe, heat 2 tablespoons extra-virgin olive oil in a medium skillet. Add Short Cooked broccoli rabe and chopped garlic to taste. Add ½ cup broth or water, cover, and cook over medium heat for 3 to 5 minutes. Uncover, add hot pepper flakes (if desired), and cook until the moisture has evaporated and the broccoli rabe is crisp-tender, about 3 minutes. The result is creamy and tender but with a nice bite.

Braising Takes 15 minutes, including Short Cooking the broccoli rabe. Using raw broccoli rabe, it takes 25 minutes and is chewier and more bitter.

Steaming Turns broccoli rabe mushy unless you watch carefully and undercook it.

Roasting Cover broccoli rabe with foil part of the time so it does not dry out. Use lots of oil.

Five Ways to Use Broccoli Rabe

Braise with pancetta

·

Steam-sauté with carrots or golden raisins

·

Make quick, meatless lasagna with broccoli rabe, precooked polenta slices,
prepared tomato sauce, and pecorino cheese

·

Cook with onions, add canned yellowfin tuna, and toss with pasta

Make a melted cheese sandwich with fontina over soft-cooked broccoli rabe

———

BROCCOLI RABE RECIPES

WHITE BEAN AND BROCCOLI RABE BRUSCHETTA

MEATBALLS WITH RED PEPPER TOMATO SAUCE

BRUSSELS SPROUTS

Brussels sprouts are not baby or miniature cabbages. Their nutritional content and health benefit are so different that Brussels sprouts and cabbage both belong on your must-eat list.

The days of abused, overcooked Brussels sprouts are over now that chefs have shown how delicious they are when they are roasted, sautéed, and even served raw. Recipes here show how to prepare them all of these ways.

Why it's good: Brussels sprouts contain an alphabet of vitamins and minerals—A, C, K, folate, riboflavin, which is essential for building body tissue, thiamine, copper to help your thyroid function, iron, magnesium, manganese, phosphorus, and potassium. They are also rich in an abundance of antioxidants, especially lutein and zeaxanthin. Containing the most sulfur-based glucosinolates of all the cruciferous vegetables gives Brussels sprouts the ability to kill more cancer cells than other crucifers. A 1-cup serving also provides 3 grams of protein and 3 grams of fiber.

What to Look For

Brussels sprouts should be medium to dark green—or purple—and feel hard, with tightly wrapped leaves. Avoid Brussels sprouts that are yellowing, spotted, cracked, smell like cabbage, or have several layers of loose outer leaves. Selecting ones around the same size helps them cook evenly.

Frozen Brussels sprouts contain far less cancer-fighting compounds. Mushy when cooked and served on their own, they are decent in soups and stews.

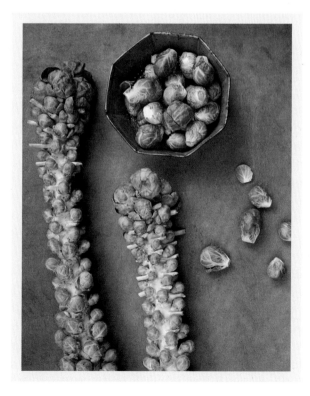

How to Buy and Store

Brussels sprouts are sold in supermarkets year-round. Farmer's markets have them from October until Christmas.

Brussels sprouts still attached to their tall stalk are often the sweetest. Release the sprouts spiraling around the stalk by cutting each sprout at its base.

Freshness predicts flavor better than size. Recently picked Brussels sprouts taste mild, even sweet. With age, they turn more bitter and dry. Big Brussels sprouts are easy to work with. Smaller ones can be more tender. Thumbnail-size ones roast beautifully.

Ten to 16 ounces of Brussels sprouts serves 4. Remember that roasting shrinks them considerably, so buy more.

Leave bagged Brussels sprouts in their container. Transfer Brussels sprouts from a net bag, plastic box, or paper container to a wide, shallow bowl, lay a paper towel over them, and cover the bowl very loosely with a plastic bag. Store the covered Brussels sprouts in the coldest part of the refrigerator. Brussels sprouts keep for up to 2 weeks, although if they start looking faded, they will taste bitter.

Basic Brussels Sprouts Techniques

WASHING

Remove the outer layer of leaves, including any that are yellowed or wilted, then rinse Brussels sprouts in a bowl of cold water.

PREPPING

Trim the bottom of sprouts but do not bother to cut an X in the bottom—it does little to help them cook evenly.

Vertically halve or quarter all but the tiniest Brussels sprouts.

To shred Brussels sprouts, halve them from base to top, then slice them crosswise.

Separating Brussels sprouts into individual leaves is time-consuming but the payoff when roasted or sautéed is outstanding.

COOKING

To steam sauté, toss with 1 or 2 tablespoons of oil. Add broth, water, or wine; cover; and cook for 5 minutes. Then cook uncovered until the liquid evaporates and the Brussels sprouts are crisp-tender.

To roast, toss halved and quartered Brussels sprouts with olive oil, coconut oil, or melted butter. Arrange them on a baking sheet in one layer, cover loosely with foil, and roast at 400°F for 15 minutes. Remove the foil, turn the sprouts cut side down, and roast 20 more minutes, until caramelized. Stir and continue to roast 10 to 20 minutes longer if you want them softer.

To steam, cook halved or quartered Brussels sprouts in a covered pot fitted with a steamer basket for 6 to 8 minutes. Toss the Brussels sprouts, hot or cooled, with the sauce used in Brussels Sprouts Pinzimonio (p. 15), or a maple mustard vinaigrette.

Brussels sprouts can be stir-fried or grilled in a grill basket.

Do not boil Brussels sprouts; they will turn an ugly olive gray color and be mushy outside while still hard inside.

To serve raw, shred Brussels sprouts finely, then massage them with oil and a bit of salt until they wilt, 3 to 5 minutes.

Five Ways to Use Brussels Sprouts

Cook Brussels sprouts in the fat from a slice of
uncured bacon, prosciutto, or pancetta

·

Toss cooked Brussels sprouts with halved green grapes and toasted walnuts

·

Mash with potatoes or sweet potatoes

·

Sauté with shallots, chopped apple, golden raisins, and dried cranberries

·

Stir-fry with smoked tofu and red bell peppers

BRUSSELS SPROUTS RECIPES

BRUSSELS SPROUTS PINZIMONIO

CABBAGE AND BRUSSELS SPROUT SOUP

BRUSSELS SPROUTS AND BROCCOLI LEAF SLAW

TOASTED COUSCOUS WITH BRUSSELS SPROUTS AND WILD MUSHROOMS

ROASTED BRUSSELS SPROUTS WITH MISO-ORANGE SPLASH

CABBAGE

Green, red, Savoy, and Napa cabbage are so different from one another that you could serve all of them at a big buffet. Red cabbage tastes sweeter than green, while Savoy is the softest, sweetest, and most elegant of these three Old World cabbages. See for yourself in Salmon Steamed in a Cabbage Leaf with Corn Butter (p. 105). Napa, aka Chinese cabbage, is truly Asian and an entirely different species. In cooking, its affinities include tofu, scallions, cilantro, ginger, miso, fermented black beans, peanuts, sesame, and soy sauce or tamari.

Why it's good: All cabbages share some health benefits but each one also has meaningful benefits of its own. All cabbage is packed with vitamins A, C, K, and folate and other B vitamins, but green cabbage has the most vitamin K, useful for the immune system. Red cabbage has three times as much antioxidant vitamin C as green. Napa has the most folate, which helps reduce the risk of birth defects during pregnancy.

All cabbages are good sources of calcium, magnesium, manganese, and other minerals. As with other crucifers, cabbages are loaded with phytochemicals. Red cabbage gets its color from anthocyanins, the same antioxidants found in red grapes and berries. Savoy cabbage has the most beta-carotene, which supports healthy skin and eyesight. It is also a particularly good source of fiber.

What to Look For

Supermarkets have these four kinds of cabbage year-round, although Savoy may disappear during the summer. Most farmer's markets have them all, too.

In fall, look particularly for heads of locally grown pointed or flattened green cabbages, heirloom varieties that are exceptionally juicy and sweet.

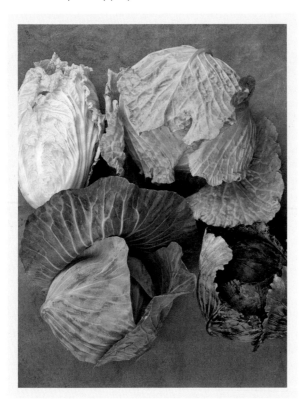

Savoy cabbage nestled in its ruff of outer leaves is nearly too beautiful to eat but its crinkled leaves are the best for stuffing and for layering in dishes.

Napa cabbage is either a barrel-shaped, chubby, and loose head or it is tall and narrow, with flattened, tightly wrapped leaves.

The outer leaves of a cabbage shelter the inner head from pesticides but organic cabbage often tastes better because of the mineral-rich soil it grows in.

How to Buy and Store

Heads of red and green cabbage should be rock-hard, with no funky smell. Avoid any that are cracked, blemished, or spotted.

Savoy cabbage is less dense but a head should feel heavy for its size. Heads around 6 inches in diameter are best.

Napa cabbage should have white, firm stems and crinkled leaves that hug the head. Some black speckling on the stems is okay. Avoid heads with spongy or flabby stems, or leaves with torn or browned edges.

All cabbage should be moist where it was cut at the bottom, not browned or dried out.

Cut cabbage quickly loses nutritional value along with flavor. Finely shredded cabbage meant for salads and slaw fares the worst. So buy a whole cabbage, or a cut half if you must.

An 8-ounce wedge of cabbage, cored and finely shredded, makes about 2½ cups. Savoy, fluffier than green or red cabbage, yields about 2 cups. A 1-pound head of Napa cabbage is perfect for most stir-fry or salad recipes when shredded, yielding 7 to 8 cups. But most heads are bigger, making this the rare time I recommend buying a cut half wrapped in plastic.

Green and red cabbage, tightly sealed in plastic wrap, keep for 2 weeks or more in the bottom of the refrigerator. Wrap Savoy cabbage in paper towels; it should keep at least one week stored in the bottom of the refrigerator. Napa, also wrapped in paper towels, keeps for 1 week. All cut heads, tightly wrapped, keep for 5 days. Use packaged shredded cabbage as soon as possible. Always store cabbage away from apples and other fruit that give off ethylene gas.

Basic Cabbage Techniques

WASHING

For a whole head, a quick rinse is fine since the outer leaves keep its inner layers clean. Rinse packaged cut cabbage to remove possible bacteria, then spin dry.

PREPPING

To quarter a head of cabbage, cut a slice off the bottom of green, red, or Savoy cabbage, stand the head on its stem end, and using a sharp, heavy knife, halve it vertically. Place each half cut side down and halve it vertically. Turn the quarters onto one side and cut away the core, keeping enough to hold the layers together.

To quarter Napa cabbage, lay the head on its side, stem end toward you. Using a cleaver or sharp, heavy knife, halve it lengthwise. Place the halves cut side down and halve them lengthwise.

SHREDDING

Using a food processor produces wet cabbage. This moisture makes for soggy salads and cabbage that steams instead of sautéing. Shredding by hand produces better results even if strips are uneven. With a bit of practice, you will shred enough cabbage in mere minutes to serve 8 or more people.

Cut cored quarters of green, red, or Savoy cabbage crosswise to the thickness you want, the thinner, the better for slaw. Stop when strips are more tough rib than tender leaf. Cut Napa into ½-inch strips. Shredded cabbage can be covered and refrigerated for 24 hours.

FOR WHOLE LEAVES TO STUFF OR LAYER

Stand a whole cabbage on its head, insert a sharp, small knife at a 45-degree angle about 1 inch away from the stem, and work it in a circle around the stem. With a Savoy cabbage, this may release a few raw, whole leaves. But it is easier to submerge the cored cabbage in a large pot of boiling water for 1 minute, then move the head to a colander, stem end up, hold it under cold running water, and remove some leaves. Slowly pry off one or two layers. Repeat to remove more layers. Shred the rest of the head for soup, slaw, or unstuffed cabbage.

COOKING

Cabbage was created to be sautéed, braised, used in soup, and in raw salads. For meltingly soft sautéed cabbage, use plenty of fat. Go lighter on oil when stir-frying.

Cabbage can also be steamed, stir-fried, roasted, or grilled. The only time it should be boiled is in soup or for a New England boiled dinner.

Most cabbages are good cooked with apples, onions, pork of any kind, carrots and other root vegetables, tomatoes, caraway seed, cumin, dill, ginger or parsley, and raisins and other dried fruits. Napa cabbage's affinities are scallions, ginger, cilantro, fermented black beans, tofu, miso, peanuts, sesame, and soy sauce or tamari.

Five Ways to Use Cabbage

Cut Napa cabbage leaves into scoop-size strips and
serve with hummus and dips

·

Grill Savoy cabbage wedges and drizzle with the liquid from kimchi

·

Add shredded Napa cabbage or red cabbage to green salads

·

Cook shredded green cabbage and onions until caramelized and toss with egg noodles

·

Sauté red or green cabbage with a chopped apple and sliced shallots

---

CABBAGE RECIPES

CABBAGE AND BRUSSELS SPROUT SOUP

THAI COCONUT SOUP WITH SHRIMP AND SAVOY CABBAGE

SALMON STEAMED IN A CABBAGE LEAF WITH CORN BUTTER

KIMCHI FRIED RICE WITH CRISPED TOFU

RED KALE, RED CABBAGE, AND DRIED CHERRIES

ROASTED CABBAGE DRIZZLED WITH GREEN HARISSA

CHARD AND BEET GREENS

Chard has meaty leaves and ribbed stems that cook up crunchy and sweet. A bunch of beets also has two edible parts—ruby roots and green leaves that look like red chard's slimmer cousin. Their mineral, earthy taste is remarkably similar to chard, which makes sense since they are related.

Chard has green leaves but its stems can be electric yellow, salmon pink, orange, magenta, or red, as well as creamy white. Chard with white stems, also called Swiss chard, tastes mildest. Yellow chard is more bitter, and red chard has the strongest flavor, with the other colors falling somewhere in between. Rainbow chard refers to bunches made up of chard in several colors. For beets, the greens look pretty much the same, no matter the color of the beets.

Chard is an excellent source of vitamins A and C, both important antioxidants. It is rich in folate, a B-vitamin that supports heart health, and it is loaded with vitamin K, which supports healthy teeth, especially together with chard's calcium content. Chard contains sky-high amounts of the carotinoids lutein and zeaxanthin. It is also a good source of iron.

Beet greens have nutritional benefits similar to those of chard.

Chard and beet greens are high in oxalic acid. If you have kidney issues, gout, or take a blood thinner, check with your doctor about eating them.

What to Look For

Chard and red chard are found at supermarkets year-round while the other kinds appear less consistently. Supermarkets also sell beets with their tops most of the year.

Chard leaves can be shiny or matte, and crinkled or fairly flat. White chard stems are tender-crisp but most of the vividly colored ones are fibrous and tough.

Buying organic is wise since conventionally grown chard can soak up nitrates from applied fertilizers that our bodies can convert into cancer-causing nitrites.

How to Buy and Store

Look for bouncy leaves and firm stems. Avoid bunches with leaves that are torn or cracked or have browned edges. Stems should be unblemished and firm.

For beet greens, select bunches of beets with abundant leaves without tears, yellowing, or brown or black spots. Red splotches or spots are okay. How dark the leaves and stems of beets are depends on the color of the beets: The darker the beets are, the deeper green their leaves and redder their stems. The palest leaves are from golden and striped Chioggia beets.

Bunches of chard weigh ½ to 1¼ pounds. The leaves may measure 24 inches from end to end, with prominent veins and wide stems, or they can be 10 inches and narrow, with a skinny stem. Individual recipes here tell how much to buy. Chard is so versatile you can toss any extra into soups, use it in a frittata, or mash it into a baked potato.

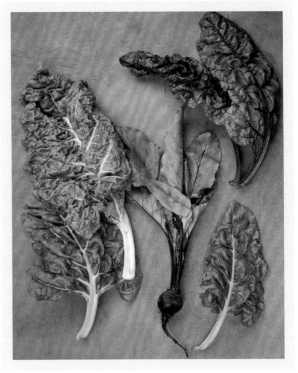

Beet greens are the bonus you get when buying a bunch of beets. The leaves of 1 bunch usually make 1 serving. For more, at local markets, ask a friendly farmer and he or she may give you additional greens since most beet buyers foolishly discard the leaves.

Chard wilts easily so get it home promptly. Immediately remove the band. If desired, cut off the stems at the base of the leaves and discard them. Or wrap the leaves and stems each loosely in paper towels and store, bottom ends out, in a loosely closed plastic bag in the crisper drawer for up to 3 days.

Beets greens keep best separated from the beets, wrapped in a paper towel and stored like chard for 2 to 3 days.

Basic Chard and Beet Green Techniques

WASHING

Wash leaves in a large bowl of cold water, paying special attention around the bottom of leaves around the stem and center vein. Empty the bowl, rinse, and repeat once or twice. Shake the leaves to remove excess water.

To remove the stem and tough center vein from chard, a V-Cut (p. 9) is best. Use Fold and Tear (p. 8) for beet greens.

COOKING

Braise, sauté, or add chard to soups and stews. It can also be steamed or stir-fried.

As it cooks, chard releases a lot of dark liquid that can make dishes look muddy. Short Cooking eliminates this. Be sure to squeeze the cooled, cooked chard well.

Chopping chard is easier after it is Short Cooked. This also helps the leaves retain more nutrients. Cook beet greens the same way as chard, alone or combined with chard, kale, or spinach. They are more tender, so Short Cook them briefly, about 2 minutes, or skip it.

Five Ways to Use Chard and Beet Greens

Sauté red chard with chickpeas and onions
and serve over whole-grain pasta

·

Stuff roasted acorn squash with garlic-sautéed chard
and top with grated Parmesan cheese

·

Top a pizza with sliced potatoes, sautéed chard, and Fontina cheese

·

Stuff a scooped-out tomato with brown rice, sautéed chard, and walnuts

·

Add beet greens to miso soup

———

CHARD AND BEET GREEN RECIPES

CAPONATA OF DARK GREENS

BLACK LENTIL SOUP WITH CHARD

BEETS AND BEET GREENS WITH CITRUS DRESSING

BLACK RICE SALAD WITH RED CHARD AND CRANBERRIES

GREEK LENTIL STEW

COD WITH ROASTED EGGPLANT RATATOUILLE

TURKEY HASH WITH SWEET POTATO AND GREENS

ITALIAN BRAISED GREENS WITH ROASTED GARLIC

CHARD WITH BROWNED ONIONS

ROASTED WINTER SQUASH WITH GINGER-BRAISED GREENS

CILANTRO

Cilantro, like James Bond, has a license to kill. In a good way, since it contains an antibacteria that scientists have proven kills salmonella. Other phytonutrients in cilantro also help it delay spoiling in foods.

Julia Child said she would throw cilantro on the floor. But hating it is limiting since Latin, Chinese, Southeast Asian, and Indian cooking all use cilantro. It is also used around the Mediterranean, in the Middle East, and parts of Africa. Eating cilantro before a meal, say in salsa or garnishing soup, stimulates the appetite. Afterward, it calms and soothes indigestion, a good thing when you eat too many tacos or too much Thai curry.

Why it's good: Eating cilantro can reduce blood pressure in people with hypertension. It reduces total cholesterol and bad LDL levels, while increasing good HDL. If this is not enough, cilantro can help rid the body of heavy metals.

Cilantro is a good source of choline, which helps efficient brain functioning, and beta-carotene, an antioxidant that helps protect the lungs. It is also a good source of vitamins A and K and a host of antioxidant phytonutrients including flavonoids like quercitin.

To enjoy cilantro's benefits, add ½ cup to smoothies, use it abundantly in salads, and spoon Red Chimichurri (p. 176) lavishly over simply cooked fish, poultry, or pork chops.

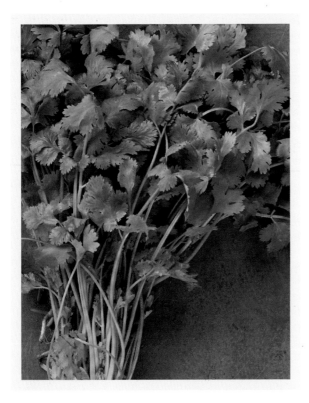

What to Look For

Cilantro is sold in supermarkets and ethnic markets year-round, and farmer's markets in season. Farmer's markets also may have feathery delfino cilantro, which looks like dill and has a milder, sweeter flavor.

Cilantro blossoms with tiny, pale pink flowers and bears small green balls. Use the flowers in salads. Dry the balls until they turn beige and you have coriander seed. This is the only plant used as both an herb and a spice.

TELLING CILANTRO FROM PARSLEY

Cilantro is also called Chinese parsley and its lacy leaves do strongly resemble flat-leaf parsley. These herbs are, in fact, botanically related, and for some people the only way to tell them apart is fragrance—released by rubbing on a leaf.

How to Buy and Store

Buy bunches with bouncy leaves and lively stems. Peer inside bunches to see if yellowed, rotting leaves or stems are lurking. Bunches where the roots are attached stay fresh longer. A small bunch is enough to provide the amount called for in most recipes.

If cilantro has roots, place it in a glass with water, cover the leaves with a paper towel, and slip a paper bag with holes punched in it over the glass. Refrigerate the covered cilantro, which will keep for up to 5 days.

For cilantro with cut stems, spread a bunch out on paper towels, roll loosely, place in a plastic bag, close loosely, and store the cilantro in the crisper drawer of the refrigerator for up to 5 days.

Basic Cilantro Techniques

WASHING

Just before using, cut away the root, if necessary, rinse sprigs in cold water, and spin them dry.

PREPPING

Cilantro sprigs have one leaf or a triple cluster at the top of the stem and a pair of leaves farther down. The stem between them is tender. Using a scissors, snip the leaves, including this fine stem, and discard the tougher stem below. Or tear or cut off the upper part and chop it, leaves and stem together.

COOKING

Cilantro can turn bitter during long cooking, so add it to dishes toward the end.

Five Ways to Use Cilantro

Combine with romaine, spinach, cucumber, pineapple, and
coconut water for a green smoothie

·

Toss with corn kernels, black beans, and jalapeño pepper for black bean salsa

·

Top grilled salmon with a pesto of cilantro, mint, shallots, and
Thai green curry paste

·

Mash with roasted eggplant and tahini

·

Mix chopped garlic, cilantro, parsley, mint, paprika, and shallots
and spoon over grilled seafood or chicken

———

COLLARD GREENS

We associate collards with the American South, but they originated around the Mediterranean. Their first road trip was to Scotland, accompanying the invading Romans. Centuries later, the Scots brought collard greens to the American South, where slaves transported from Africa began using collards to replace greens they had known at home. During the Great Migration of blacks from the South in the twentieth century, they took collard greens north and west, including to California. Meanwhile, in Europe collard greens made it to Slavic areas and via Spain to Portugal. The Portuguese brought them to Brazil, while moving in the opposite direction, collard greens recrossed the Atlantic to Africa and on to India. Collard Greens Cacciatore (p. 159), Coconut Rice with Black Beans and Collard Greens (p. 140), and Collard Green Dolmas Filled with Wild Rice and Sun-Dried Tomato Pesto (p. 33) reflect these world travels.

Why it's good: Collard greens are rich in vitamins A, C, K, B-6, which supports the nervous system, folate, and magnesium, which is important for maintaining strong bones, as well as potassium, which helps the body maintain proper acid-alkaline balance, beta-carotene, lutein, and zeaxanthin. They contain enough calcium to be called the green cow. Like the other crucifers, they contain phytochemicals that help detoxify and protect against the effects of toxins as well as isothiocyanates, sulfur compounds that help prevent and fight cancers.

Collard greens, in addition, contain tryptophan, the amino acid associated with promoting sleep. The 5 grams of protein in a cup of cooked collard greens make meatless Red Beans and Smoky Greens (p. 91) and Coconut Rice with Black Beans and Collard Greens (p. 140) substantial dishes.

What to Look For

Collard greens are sold in supermarkets and natural food stores year-round. You will find them at local farmer's markets mainly from May to November. The best are 8 to 12 inches long, supple, with an even green color and unblemished stems. Avoid leaves that are wilted, yellowing, torn, or have slimy patches.

Collard greens are naturally pest resistant, but remember that organic farming is good for the land and clean water, not only to avoid chemical residue on foods.

How to Buy and Store

You will find collard greens sold in bunches, sometimes with the leaves attached to a thick central stem. They are priced by the pound or by the bunch. A bunch can be a 1½-pound armload of elephant ear–size greens or a skimpy 8 ounces made up of 5 leaves barely larger than your hand. Chopped collard greens are sold in 16-ounce bags.

Collared leaves can be thin and flexible or thick and leathery. This makes figuring out the servings in a bunch easier based on weight than by measuring raw collards in cups. Collards cook down less than kale or mustard greens. A 12-ounce bunch of collard greens yields 1½ cups cooked.

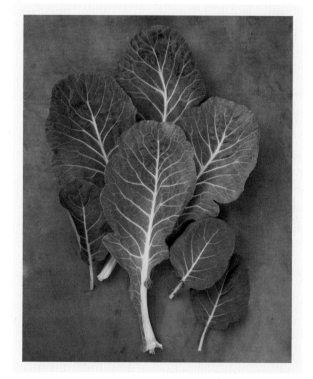

At home, remove any ties or banding. Wrap the bunch loosely in paper towels and slip the collard greens into a plastic bag, stem ends toward the opening. Keep the bag loosely closed. Store collard greens in the coldest part of the refrigerator for 3 days, keeping them away from apples or other produce that gives off ethylene gas, which hastens yellowing.

Basic Collard Green Techniques

WASHING

Collard greens can be sandy. Fill a large bowl with cold water and swish whole leaves in it. Drain, rinse the bowl, and repeat. Shake and drain the leaves. If you are Short Cooking or steaming collards, leave them damp; otherwise blot them dry with paper towels.

Always rinse bagged collard greens, which are more likely to be contaminated with bacteria than loose bunches.

STRIPPING

Collard stems and the center vein of the leaf are tough and should be removed. If leaves are flexible enough to fold and are 12 inches or less from leaf top to stem tip, use the Fold and Tear technique (p. 8). For very large or leathery collard greens, use the V-Cut (p. 9).

Bags of chopped collard greens include stem pieces. Dump the contents into a colander and pick through them. Discard pieces that are only stem. If the stem ends are brown or dry, cut off a thin slice.

CUTTING AND CHOPPING

For neatly sliced collard greens, separate stripped leaves into two long halves. Stack three or four halves that are roughly the same size. Roll the leaves lengthwise into a long tube. With a sharp knife, cut the leaves crosswise into ½-inch to ¾-inch strips. After cooking, you can chop the long ribbons to make squares and rectangles.

Alternatively, you can chop collard greens after they are cooked. This preserves more of their nutrient value and is also easier. Simply chop the drained greens.

COOKING

Short Cooking and Quick Cooling makes collard greens that are chewy-tender. It reduces the cooking time for finished dishes and avoids soups and casseroles that look murky because of juices released by raw collard greens.

Braise, steam, or roast collard greens until crisp (p. 178).

Five Ways to Use Collard Greens

Garnish lentil soup with a topknot of
Short Cooked collard greens

·

Mash steamed collard greens with roasted sweet potato

·

Stew collard greens with a smoked turkey wing

·

Make a soup with chopped collard greens, pink kidney beans, and green bell pepper

·

Sauté finely shredded collard leaves with baby carrots and ginger

COLLARD GREENS RECIPES

COLLARD GREEN DOLMAS FILLED WITH WILD RICE
AND SUN-DRIED TOMATO PESTO

ROASTED TOMATO SOUP WITH CRISPED COLLARD GREENS

KALE

Kale still tops the list of super-charged greens, along with broccoli leaves and collard greens. All of them provide potent protection thanks to phytochemicals they contain, in addition to an abundance of essential vitamins and minerals. Kale even offers useful amounts of protein and fiber. If you already love kale, bravo! If not, here are recipes that can change your mind, from kale cooked with olive oil and garlic until it melts, to egg or pasta dishes, salads, and a pesto made with raw kale. Pickled kale stems are terrific. So is crunchy roasted kale in a surprising trail mix.

Serving kale often is easy because it comes in more varieties than other dark, leafy greens. Supermarkets and natural food stores sell curly and Tuscan kale in bunches and packages of it chopped, alone, and in blends of salad greens, for cooking, or as baby leaves. Farmer's markets have as many as eight kinds of kale in season.

Why it's good: Kale contains some of the highest amounts of phytochemicals found in brassicas, including glucosinolates, which help detoxify and protect against the effects of carcinogenic toxins around us, and substances protecting us from the estrogenic effect of chemicals that promote storing belly fat. It is a good source of vitamins A, C, and K, several B vitamins, and carotenoids. The minerals in kale, including calcium, manganese, magnesium, and potassium, help to maintain your muscles, balance your metabolism, and reduce the risk of type-2 diabetes. A 1-cup serving provides 3 grams of fiber and 3 grams of protein.

What to Look For

Supermarkets and natural food markets sell at least green curly kale and Tuscan kale year-round. At local farmer's markets look for as many as eight kinds of kale, particularly between May and November. Because of pesticide residues found on conventionally grown kale, buying organic is a good choice.

CURLY KALE

This ruffle-edged kale with medium-green to dark blue-green leaves is sold nearly everywhere. You also find it in dark garnet red, especially at natural food stores and farmer's markets. Curly kale may be tough and taste bitter when fully grown, especially during warm weather, but smaller leaves will be more tender and sweet. Being hit by a late fall frost adds sweetness, too. Cook curly kale or use it raw in salads and smoothies.

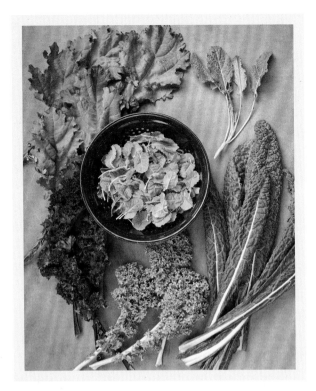

TUSCAN KALE

It is also called lacinato, cavolo nero, and even dino kale because the crinkly surface of its spear-shaped, black-green leaves supposedly resembles dinosaur skin. This chefs' favorite is an antique heirloom variety that turns meltingly tender when cooked long and slow. Supermarkets and most natural food stores sell it year-round.

Cook Tuscan kale or use it raw in salads.

RUSSIAN KALE

This mild-tasting variety has feathery, tender leaves that can be grayish to silvery green, reminiscent of the color of olive leaves. Winter frost turns its veins red-purple and tinges the leaves dusty purple. There is also red Russian kale. Russian kale is rarely seen in supermarkets but is often sold at farmer's markets and in natural food stores. It is sometimes called Siberian kale. It is a good starter if you are not a kale eater.

Russian kale is good cooked, not raw.

BABY KALE

Baby kale is chewy yet tender and mild tasting. It has all the goodness of mature kale. This is the easiest kale to use. It comes in plastic boxes and in bags containing leaves of one variety or a combination of kinds and colors.

Baby kale, perfect in salads and smoothies, can also be cooked.

ORNAMENTAL OR FLOWERING KALE

Sold in sunburst-shaped heads in shades of rose to purple, or cream and pale green, this decorative kale is tough and does not taste great, so stick to enjoying it for its looks.

How to Buy and Store

Select bunches with erect stems and firm leaves. Avoid flabby stems and yellowing, bruised, or wilted leaves. Tiny holes in organic kale leaves caused by insects do not affect the taste.

Chopped kale sold in plastic boxes and bags is convenient but inspect them and avoid packages showing dried or browned stem ends or too many chunks of stem.

Kale yellows in 3 to 4 days. If you cannot use it in time, Short Cook and then freeze it. Defrosted, it is ready to make Italian Braised Greens with Roasted Garlic (p. 145) or to toss into soup or a casserole.

Kale collapses a lot as it cooks. An 8-ounce bunch of curly kale cooks down to 1 to 1½ cups. Tuscan and Russian kale collapse even more, with an 8-ounce bunch yielding 1 cup cooked.

At home, remove any banding. Place kale in a plastic bag, stem end toward the opening. Add a paper towel to absorb moisture. Keep the bag loosely closed. Store kale in the coldest part of the refrigerator.

Store it away from apples or other produce that gives off ethylene gas, which hastens yellowing.

Basic Kale Techniques

WASHING

Rinse whole leaves under cold running water or swish them in a large bowl of water. Shake to remove excess water, or pat dry with paper towels. Always rinse bagged kale, which is more susceptible to bacteria than bunches.

PREPPING

Stripping Kale's stem becomes a tough center vein running up the leaf. It also tastes bitter. Remove it with the Fold and Tear technique (p. 8) or use the V-Cut (p. 9) on kale leaves that lie flat.

For baby kale, ignore the short stem or tear it off at the base of the leaf.

Bagged kale may include tough pieces of stem. Dump it into a colander, pick out the stem pieces, and tear leafy parts away if pieces are mostly stem, then wash the kale.

Add thinly sliced curly kale stems to Quinoa Pilaf with Carrot and Kale Stems (p. 132) or pickle them in Impatient Piccalilli (p. 181). Use a few stems when juicing. Stems from other kinds of kale are too tough to use.

Slicing and Shredding Short Cooking whole leaves of kale before chopping them is easiest and it preserves more of their nutrients.

When you want kale cut in ribbons, pull deveined leaves apart into two long halves. Stack two or three halves around the same size and roll them into a long tube. Do not worry if it is loose and unkempt. Using a sharp knife, cut the leaves crosswise into thin strips or wider ribbons. For salads, finely shredded kale is best. For cooked dishes, ½-inch to ¾-inch strips are good.

Massaging For salads, massaging raw kale breaks down the fiber, so it is chewy rather than tough. In a large bowl, drizzle oil onto chopped kale. Work the kale with your fingers until it is shiny, limp, and looks darker, which takes a few minutes. Massaging works especially well on curly and Tuscan kale.

COOKING

Braising is the most delicious way to cook kale; it is good with all varieties, most of all Tuscan kale. Short Cooking it before braising reduces total cooking time and the result is kale that's even more tender and milder tasting.

Short Cooking Short Cooked kale can be seasoned and served as is if you like it on the chewy side, or sautéed, braised, or added to soups, stews, cooked grains, beans, and other dishes. It cooks more quickly and saves time overall. Short Cook kale until almost tender, 3 to 4 minutes, or until very tender, 7 to 10 minutes. Immediately Quick Cool it. For instructions, see p. 7.

Steaming produces chewy kale with clear flavor. It works best with green curly kale. Place a steamer insert into a large pot. Add 1 to 2 inches of water, cover, and bring to a boil. Add the raw leaves, either whole or cut up. Steam, covered, until the kale collapses, about 5 minutes. Immediately Quick Cool steamed kale to set the color and avoid mushy texture.

Serve steamed kale as is, or sauté, braise, or add to soups, stews, cooked grains, beans, and other dishes.

Always squeeze excess moisture from cooked kale. This takes time and patience but it is essential for good texture and to avoid dishes that are watery—even when kale will go into a soup.

Five Ways to Use Kale

Place pan-seared turkey cutlets on a bed of cooked kale and
deglaze the pan with apple cider for a sauce

·

Top crostini of smoked mozzarella with braised kale and chopped tomatoes

·

Toss chopped Tuscan kale, sun-dried tomatoes,
and corn with whole-wheat macaroni

·

Steam green curly kale and butternut squash, and serve with short-grain brown rice

·

Crumble Crisped Kale into chocolate chip cookie dough

KALE RECIPES

KALE PESTO WITH CARROT AND SWEET PEPPER CRUDITÉS

CAYENNE SHORTBREAD WITH CRISPED KALE

ROASTED RED PEPPERS STUFFED WITH KALE

RIBBOLITA WITH TUSCAN KALE

ROOT VEGETABLE CHOWDER WITH KALE

TUSCAN KALE SALAD WITH POMEGRANATE SEEDS AND WALNUTS

BABY KALE AND TUNA SALAD WITH GRAPE TOMATOES, SWEET ONION,
AND WASABI DRESSING

TURKEY AND KALE SALAD WITH CRANBERRIES AND CIDER DRESSING

TURKEY HASH WITH SWEET POTATO AND GREENS

KALE-SMOTHERED PORK CHOPS WITH CARROT AND APPLE

FUSILLI WITH CHICKPEAS AND TUSCAN KALE

QUINOA PILAF WITH CARROT AND KALE STEMS

ITALIAN BRAISED GREENS WITH ROASTED GARLIC

TUSCAN KALE WITH RAISINS AND PINE NUTS

KALE COLCANNON

MUSTARD-GLAZED GREEN KALE

RED KALE, RED CABBAGE, AND DRIED CHERRIES

KALE ZA'ATAR

CRISPED KALE, COLLARD GREENS, OR BROCCOLI LEAF

IMPATIENT PICCALILLI

POACHED EGG IN A NEST OF BACON-WILTED KALE

DILL-PICKLED KALE STEMS

POWER OATMEAL

OATMEAL EVERYTHING COOKIES

CHOCOLATE FUDGE ENERGY BOMBS

POPCORN TRAIL MIX

MUSTARD GREENS

The heat and bitterness of mustard greens challenge our American palate, so here are recipes that gentle them. These versions of soul food favorites and Indian dishes let you enjoy mustard greens while keeping intact more of the life-preserving phytochemicals responsible for their strong taste.

Why it's good: The mustard greens I use are the bright green, bouffant kind sometimes called Southern or American mustard greens. Their frilly lime green leaves get their bite from sulfur-based compounds that help cleanse the liver by neutralizing toxins. The bitterness also comes from isothiocyanates, indoles, and other phytonutrients found in most brassicas. Mustard greens contain antioxidants like vitamins A, C, and K that bolster your immune system, as well. They are rich in magnesium, good for nerves and bones, and calcium. Plus you get 2 grams of protein and 2 grams of fiber in a cup of cooked mustard greens.

What to Look For

Supermarkets and natural food stores sell Southern or American mustard greens year-round. Farmer's markets usually have them from May through November. These greens may also be garnet red or beet purple. The red varieties are tougher and may be hairy but taste the same as green ones.

How to Buy and Store

Select mustard greens with lively leaves. Avoid any that are limp, yellowing, have slimy spots or browned edges, or tears, especially around any banding. Mustard greens wilt quickly so get them home promptly.

Bunches weigh 8 to 20 ounces. They also come in 10- and 16-ounce bags.

Chopped, these greens appear in packaged stir-fry and braising blends. Baby mustard greens are used in micro-blends.

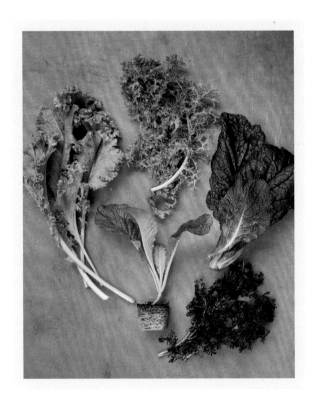

Mustard greens collapse a lot, and a 12-ounce bunch or 1-pound bag cooks down to 1¼ cups.

At home, remove any banding. Wrap the leaves in paper towels and slip mustard greens into a plastic bag, stem ends toward the opening. Keep the bag loosely closed. Store mustard greens in the crisper drawer of the refrigerator for up to 3 days.

Store them away from apples or other produce that give off ethylene gas.

Basic Mustard Greens Techniques

WASHING

Just before cooking, wash whole leaves in a large bowl of cold water. They can be sandy, so swish them vigorously, paying particular attention to rippling folds and the backs of leaves. Empty the bowl, rinse, and repeat once or twice. Shake the leaves to eliminate excess moisture. Leave mustard greens damp if Short Cooking or steaming them. Otherwise blot them dry with paper towels.

Always wash bagged mustard greens, which are more likely to be contaminated with bacteria than loose bunches.

PREPPING

Stripping Mustard greens stems are fibrous, so remove them and the vein running up the center of the leaf as well. Because of their billowing shape, the Fold and Tear technique (p. 8) works best. With packaged chopped mustard greens, discard pieces that are mainly stem.

Chopping Mustard greens discolor at cut edges, so Quick Cook or steam them whole, then chop them before further cooking. To chop raw mustard greens, roll a leaf into a rough tube and cut it crosswise into strips. Pile the strips and coarsely chop them.

COOKING

Four cooking methods work with mustard greens, depending on how mild-tasting and tender you want them.

My favorite is mustard greens Short Cooked for 3 to 4 minutes, then Quick Cooled. The result is pleasantly sharp and still chewy, ready for sautéing, braising, or adding to stews, soups, or stir-fries. If not using them immediately, refrigerate in a covered container for up to 3 days.

Sautéing Short Cooked–Quick Cooled chopped mustard greens in peanut, coconut, olive, or cold-pressed sesame oil for about 5 minutes makes greens with good body and comfortably sharp flavor.

Steaming mustard greens for about 6 minutes produces a similar effect.

Five Ways to Use Mustard Greens

Braise shredded mustard greens in coconut milk
with curry powder and serve over rice

·

Simmer chopped Short Cooked mustard greens with
chunks of daikon radish, carrot, shiitake mushrooms, and miso

·

Mash braised mustard greens with roasted butternut squash and scallions

·

Stew Short Cooked mustard greens with chopped tomato, onion, and leek

·

Mix Short Cooked mustard greens into Vietnamese pho

PARSLEY

Call it an herb but eat parsley like a vegetable. Truly notice parsley's clean flavor and you will enjoy using it liberally, as Mediterranean and Middle Eastern cooks do in Zucchini, Onion, and Fresh Herb Frittata (p. 191) and in Red Quinoa Tabbouleh (p. 77) made with more greens than grain. Condiments, including Green Harissa (p. 168) and Italian Salsa Verde (p. 15), are more piquant ways to add parsley when you serve grilled chicken, seafood, tofu, or vegetables.

Science has demonstrated that parsley's combination of vitamins A, C, K, and folate, potassium, iron, an abundance of carotenoids, and the phytonutrients myrsitcin, which helps neutralize carcinogens, and luteolin, an antioxidant that helps increase the blood's oxygen capacity, provides two kinds of benefits. It is detoxifying, which helps to prevent tumors from forming. In addition, substances in parsley fight inflammation associated with heart disease, asthma, arthritis, and other chronic diseases. Eating parsley can help to control blood pressure and blood sugar levels, too.

What to Look For

There are two kinds of parsley: the flat-leaf, also called Italian parsley, and curly parsley. Supermarkets sell both kinds year-round.

FLAT-LEAF

Flat clearly describes the fernlike dark green leaves of Italian parsley. A fresh bunch is so perky that I sometimes set it in a jar of ice water on the counter as a kitchen bouquet. Use flat-leaf parsley in dishes, raw or cooked, saving curly parsley for decoration. Its deeper color says flat-leaf parsley is nutritionally intense, plus it tastes sweeter than curly parsley. Add it as full sprigs to soups, stews, stock, and broth; use whole leaves in salads; or chop and add it to all kinds of dishes, from soups and stews to pasta dishes.

CURLY PARSLEY

Its bouncy tufts look nice as a garnish and hold up better than flat-leaf sprigs. But this ruffled variety tastes bitter and feels prickly and tough when you eat it. It is also harder to work under your knife for chopping.

How to Buy and Store

Parsley should have firm stems and erect leaves. Avoid bunches with pale, yellowing, or wilted leaves or limp stems. Tiny holes or dry brown spots on organic parsley leaves may be caused by insects; they do not affect the taste. Buying organic lets you avoid possible residue from chemicals used to control mildew, fungus, or weeds. Bunches weigh 2 to 4 ounces. A 4-ounce bunch yields out 1 cup of stemmed, chopped flat-leaf parsley. Since parsley can last for more than a week, select the biggest bunch.

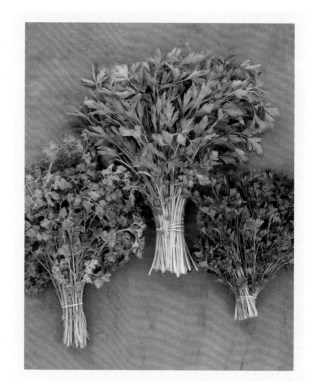

At home, remove any banding. Discard sprigs with bruised leaves and any that are yellowed or limp. Separate out short-stemmed sprigs and set them aside to use first.

For storing, there are two schools of thought. Some people wrap parsley in a paper towel and place it, stem end out, in a loosely closed plastic bag in the refrigerator's vegetable crisper, where it should keep for up to 5 days. Others place the bunch in a glass, add an inch or two of water, lay a folded paper towel on top of the parsley, and set a plastic bag loosely over the parsley. Occasionally, lift off the bag, turn it inside out, give it a good shake, and set it loosely back over the parsley. I find parsley kept this way lasts up to 10 days. Be careful not to knock over the glass! Store parsley away from apples and other fruits that give off ethylene gas.

Wilted parsley perks up nicely when refrigerated in a bowl of ice water for an hour.

Basic Parsley Techniques

WASHING

Cut off the stems of whole sprigs or pluck the leaves, then swish parsley in a bowl of cold water and spin dry.

PLUCKING PARSLEY

Only chefs and obsessive cooks pluck parsley one leaf at a time, making sure no stem is attached. These following methods work much faster.

For Flat-Leaf Parsley Holding a group of sprigs together, pull down on their stems until the lowest leaves line up. Lay the bouquet horizontally on a cutting board, and with a large, sharp knife cut off the stems just below the leaves. With your fingers, pluck out the toughest bits of stem.

To eliminate more stem, hold a sprig in one hand. With your other hand, bring the lower leaves and top cluster of leaves together and tear them off the stem. This method is slower but more precise. Discard the stems or save them. They will keep for a week, wrapped in a paper towel and stored in a plastic bag in your refrigerator.

Curly Parsley The leaves on curly parsley cluster near the top of the stem. Grab the top and side clusters and pull them all off together.

MEASURING PARSLEY

To get the called-for amount, see How Much Is a Cup? (p. 9). In recipes calling for "parsley, chopped," first measure the parsley, then chop it.

CHOPPING

For instant chopped parsley, hold a few sprigs over a salad or cooking pot and snip the leaves with a scissors. Along with the parsley leaves, bits of stem falling into the bowl or pot are fine.

For larger amounts, mound plucked leaves on a small cutting board and chop by rocking the blade of a large, sharp knife back and forth over them. Rotate the board 90 degrees or push the parsley together with your hands and repeat mounding, rotating, and chopping until the parsley has the fineness you want.

COOKING

Add whole sprigs or stems to broths, stews, soups, or tomato sauce. Tie them with kitchen twine so the limp sprigs are easily removed.

In hot dishes, add chopped parsley at the end to preserve its color and nutrients.

Raw parsley can be tough. For dishes using it in quantity, like Red Quinoa Tabbouleh (p. 77), letting it sit a while allows the acid in them to tenderize the parsley.

Five Ways to Use Parsley

Include chopped parsley in spaghetti aglio e olio

·

Add parsley to lentil salad with celery, red onion, and red wine vinegar

·

Toss whole leaves with mesclun and add them to mixed green salads

·

Add chopped parsley to coleslaw

·

Sprinkle chopped parsley and a drizzle of olive oil over
steamed carrots, zucchini, or string beans

PARSLEY RECIPES

BRUSSELS SPROUTS PINZIMONIO·

HUMMUS WITH ARUGULA AND PARSLEY

SHRIMP WITH GREEN HERB MAYONNAISE

ROSEMARY WALNUT PESTO

ROOT VEGETABLE CHOWDER WITH KALE

SPINACH GAZPACHO WITH WALNUTS

RED QUINOA TABBOULEH

FARRO SALAD WITH FETA AND GREEN OLIVES

MEATBALLS WITH RED PEPPER TOMATO SAUCE

INCENDIARY HERBED BROWN RICE

GARLIC AND PARSLEY MASHED POTATOES

ROASTED CABBAGE DRIZZLED WITH GREEN HARISSA

SALSA VERDE

ZUCCHINI, ONION, AND FRESH HERB FRITTATA

APPLE-PARSLEY TISANE

PARSLEY-GINGER LEMONADE

PARSLEY ELIXIR

ROMAINE LETTUCE

Iceberg lettuce is popular for its succulent crunch. Romaine lettuce equals this crispness when you include its juicy ribs. Its leaves bring you far better nutrition than iceberg and other lettuces.

Exposure to sun, pests, and disease stimulates romaine lettuce to produce substances that protect it. Heads that are open and loose, leaving more leaves vulnerable, produce more of these substances, which are the phytochemicals that are good for us, too. So rather than using only hearts of romaine, with their sheltered inner leaves, choose full heads that are loose and open to get more of romaine lettuce's benefits.

Why it's good: Romaine lettuce is an excellent source of vitamins A, C, K, and folate, and of the minerals manganese and chromium, both important for maintaining normal blood sugar levels. It provides good amounts of calcium and phosphorus. Eating 2 cups of romaine's darker outer leaves delivers more vitamin A and twice the vitamin K than the recommended daily value, nearly half the vitamin C, and a third of the amount of folate recommended. You also get carotenoids, including lutein and zeaxanthin. Romaine lettuce is also a useful source of tryptophan, the amino acid that helps promote sleep.

Lettuce ranks number fifteen on The Environmental Working Group's list of produce analyzed for pesticide residues, so you may want to buy organic.

What to Look For

Supermarkets sell romaine lettuce in heads and packaged hearts year-round. Baby romaine leaves come in plastic boxes, combined in salad mixes, or solo. Farmer's markets feature mature and baby romaine as long as the

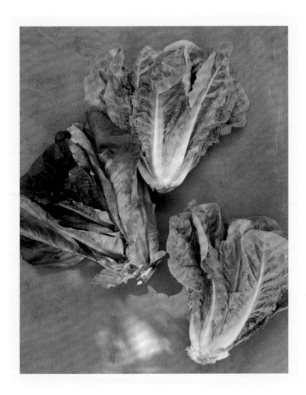

local weather permits. Some of them also have romaine lettuce with red-tipped leaves or heads with radicchio-red outer leaves and red-to-green inner leaves.

How to Buy and Store

Look for heads that feel heavy for their size and preferably fan out in shape. Leaves should be intensely green, even dark and dull-looking at the top, with ribs that are firm, succulent, and pale green. Avoid heads with torn or bruised leaves or brown, slimy spots. Avoid heads with rust-colored, bruised, or cracked ribs. Be sure the base of a head looks moist and is not cracked.

A good-size head of romaine lettuce weighs about 1 pound. A 12-inch outer leaf, including its rib or three to four inner leaves, torn into bite-size pieces, makes 1 packed cup. A whole head makes Caesar salad for 8 to 10 people.

At home, remove any banding. Wrap the head loosely in paper towels and store it, cut end out, in a loosely closed plastic bag in the crisper drawer of the refrigerator. Or deconstruct the head, arranging the leaves side by side on a very long length of paper toweling, then loosely roll it up. Store the roll in a large, loosely closed plastic bag. Either way, the lettuce will last up to a week.

Store romaine away from apples and fruits that give off ethylene gas, which turns the ribs rust red

Basic Romaine Techniques

WASHING

Just before using, separate and rinse the leaves under cold running water to remove possible bacteria as well as grit near the base of the leaves. Shake the leaves, then pat dry or tear the rinsed leaves and spin-dry.

PREPPING

Tearing Versus Cutting The edges of torn leaves discolor less. If you need shredded lettuce, stack several leaves and use a sharp knife to slice them into strips.

COOKING

Lightly cooked romaine lettuce tastes nutty. French Lettuce Stir-Fry (p. 166) and Grilled Romaine Lettuce with Beefsteak Tomatoes and Ranch Dressing (p. 65) show how good it is.

Add tough outer leaves to vegetable stock for fuller flavor.

Five Ways to Use Romaine Lettuce

Use small inner leaves to scoop up dips

·

Wrap a burger, a tomato slice, and an onion slice in a large romaine leaf

·

Juice with apple, celery, watercress, and cucumber

·

Toss shredded romaine, wakame sea vegetable, sun-dried tomatoes,
and cucumber with soy-ginger dressing

·

Whirl up a smoothie with romaine lettuce, avocado, celery,
fresh basil, coconut water, and lime juice

ROMAINE LETTUCE RECIPES

CAESAR SALAD WITH PARMESAN CHICKPEAS

GRILLED ROMAINE LETTUCE WITH BEEFSTEAK TOMATOES
AND RANCH DRESSING

SPINACH

Spinach, perhaps the most versatile Power Green, is good raw or cooked. You can use it in meatloaf, green salads, soups, and smoothies even without consulting a recipe. Using baby spinach on sandwiches is another easy choice. Spinach is also good in Tahini Creamed Spinach (p. 147) and Spinach and Cheddar Scones (p. 200). Frozen spinach, perhaps the ultimate green convenience food, is a reliable way to always have spinach on hand.

Why it's good: Spinach is an excellent source of vitamins A, C, and K. It is rich in B vitamins, especially folate, which reduces the risk of heart disease and is important for women who might become pregnant. It is a good source of minerals, particularly bone-protecting calcium, and iron.

Besides having hefty amounts of beta-carotene, lutein, and zeaxanthin, carotenoids that support healthy skin and eyes, a study on adult women showed eating spinach was inversely related to incidence of breast cancer. It also contains carotenoids that appear to protect against the most aggressive form of prostate cancer. Since your body gets different benefits from eating spinach raw or cooked, eat it both ways.

Spinach is high in oxalic acid. If you have kidney issues, gout, or take a blood thinner, check with your doctor about eating it.

What to Look For

Supermarkets carry deep green Savoy spinach, brighter green flat-leaf spinach, and tender baby spinach year-round. Farmer's markets often have spinach only in spring and again after the weather cools since spinach bolts during hot weather.

Savoy spinach, with its dark green, crinkled, meaty leaves and fibrous stems, is best used in cooked dishes. Look for it in bags or banded in bunches.

Flat-leaf spinach has spade-shaped, erect leaves and thin stems. It is good raw and cooked, where you want tender leaves with some body and milder taste than Savoy. It is sold in bunches.

Baby spinach, actually leaves picked one or two weeks before maturity, is a healthy convenience food. Use its oval leaves raw in salads, on sandwiches, or on pizza. It is so tender you can mix raw baby spinach, whole or chopped, into hot soups, omelets, and other dishes, and enjoy it just wilted. It is sold in 5-ounce boxes or bags, and loose by the pound.

Semi-Savoy spinach with lightly crinkled leaves falls between Savoy and flat-leaf spinach in meaty firmness and in color.

Spinach is heavily sprayed and listed as one of the Environmental Working Group's *Dirty Dozen,* so I buy organic.

How to Buy and Store Spinach

Spinach leaves should have even color and crisp, firm stems. Check bunches for wilting, yellowed, or torn leaves, especially around the band and in the center of bunches. Avoid spinach with curled or dry, brown stem ends. Inspect packaged spinach for bad leaves, particularly at the bottom of the bag or box.

For salads, a 5-ounce package, 4 ounces of loose baby spinach, or an 8-ounce bunch of flat-leaf spinach makes 6 servings. Spinach collapses drastically when cooked. A 5-ounce bag of baby spinach, and an 8-ounce bunch of flat-leaf spinach, stemmed, yield 1 to 1¼ cups when steamed or sautéed, which is two servings. A 10-ounce bag of Savoy spinach sautéed or braised serves just two.

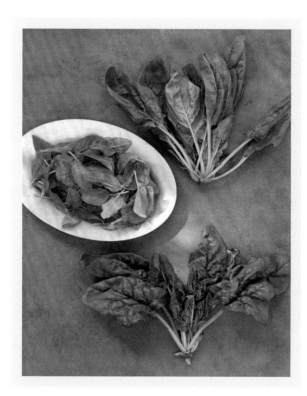

Refrigerate packaged spinach in the crisper drawer, where it will keep for three days. Immediately remove the banding on bunches. Then place the spinach in a glass with two inches of water, set a paper towel on top of the spinach, drape a plastic bag loosely over this, and refrigerate for up to three days. Or, spread the spinach out on paper toweling, roll it up loosely, and store in a loosely closed plastic bag in the crisper drawer of the refrigerator. Keep all spinach away from apples and other produce emitting ethylene gas.

Basic Spinach Cooking Techniques

WASHING

Stem and wash spinach just before using. Leave the stems of baby spinach and flat-leaf spinach or pinch them off. Use Fold and Tear to remove the tough stems from Savoy spinach.

Baby spinach needs only a rinse in a bowl of cold water. Flat-leaf and Savoy spinach require thorough washing to avoid grinding grit in your teeth. In a large bowl of cold water, swish the leaves well, then transfer them to a colander. Empty, rinse, and refill the bowl, repeating until no sand or dirt collects in the bottom of the bowl. Shake the leaves lightly and cook with the water clinging to the leaves, or spin-dry spinach for salads, stir-fries, and sautés.

PREPPING

Chopping Gather stemmed fresh spinach by the handful and cut it crosswise into strips or chop it using a sharp knife. Or snip the spinach with scissors. Holding it over the pot to add to soups and stews is a neat cook's tip.

Stems from Savoy spinach are good cut into 1-inch pieces and stir-fried together with the leaves. If you get Savoy spinach in clusters, the base, including the pink root tip, is delightfully crunchy—include it in stir-fries.

COOKING

Cooked spinach, fresh or frozen, holds water tenaciously, so squeeze right after Short Cooking or steaming and also squeeze it a second time just before sautéing, stir-frying, or adding it to a recipe. It holds so much water that squeezing it twice is the way to avoid watery lasagna or quiche and runny meatloaf or omelets.

Frozen spinach has been blanched before freezing, so you can defrost and add it directly to a dish or cook it in a splash of water. Alway squeeze it dry before using it.

To cook fresh spinach, sautéing it in oil gives the best taste and texture. These are recommended cooking times. Remember they will vary depending on the amount and kind of spinach:

Short Cook for 15 to 30 seconds

Steam for 2 minutes to wilt, 4 to 6 minutes to cook

Sauté for 5 to 8 minutes

Stir-fry for 3 to 5 minutes

Five Ways to Use Spinach

Mix chopped raw spinach into a baked potato or freshly cooked rice

·

Scramble eggs with chopped spinach

·

Toss a handful of baby spinach leaves on top of pizza

·

Mix chopped spinach into hummus

·

Make tabbouleh with chopped spinach, cherry tomatoes,
parsley, and cilantro

SPINACH RECIPES

MEXICAN SEVEN LAYER DIP

SPINACH GAZPACHO WITH WALNUTS

SPINACH SALAD WITH SEARED NECTARINES AND HONEY MUSTARD DRESSING

TOFU PICCATA WITH SAUTÉED SPINACH

BAKED MACARONI AND CHEESE WITH SPINACH

GREEN FETTUCCINI WITH SPINACH HEMP PESTO

ITALIAN BRAISED GREENS WITH ROASTED GARLIC

TAHINI CREAMED SPINACH

TURKEY SLIDERS

SPINACH AND CORN PANCAKES WITH LIME DRIZZLE

SPINACH AND CHEDDAR SCONES

ROASTED WINTER SQUASH WITH GINGER-BRAISED GREENS

WATERCRESS

Forget about serving watercress only in tea sandwiches or as a garnish. This sharp green contains so many essential vitamins, minerals, and phytonutrients, and in such abundance, that it should be used in good amounts in everyday dishes like Spicy Chopped Salad (p. 71) and livening up Glorious Greens Juice (p. 217).

Why it's good: Watercress contains more than fifteen vitamins and minerals, including A, C, E, and K (one cup provides the day's entire recommended amount of this multifunctional vitamin). It also provides good amounts of folate, riboflavin and thiamine, pantothenic acid, calcium, copper, magnesium, manganese, phosphorus, and potassium. Nitrates in watercress help maintain healthy blood pressure while alpha-lipoic acid, an antioxidant, helps your body repair damaged DNA. Chlorophyll in watercress helps block the effect of carcinogens formed when you grill foods, a good thing in Bangkok Beef Salad (p. 87) and on top of grilled burgers. Like other greens in the brassica family, watercress gets its hot and bitter flavors from an array of anti-inflammatory antioxidants and detoxifying substances. You get all this for just four calories per cup.

GREEN WATERCRESS

Nearly every supermarket sells watercress in bags or bunches. Bagged watercress is hydroponically grown. It has thin, tender stems and a paler color compared to watercress in bunches.

The watercress at farmer's markets is leggier, with curving stems. It tastes very sharp and may be wild.

RED WATERCRESS

Maroon-edged or purple leaves with green veins and green stems make this richly colored watercress easy to spot. Its fibrous stems sport round and pointed leaves. Scientists have yet to confirm whether the phytochemicals that make it red also add significantly to its nutrition.

Red watercress was discovered growing wild in Florida. What is sold today is grown from seeds originating from that wild find.

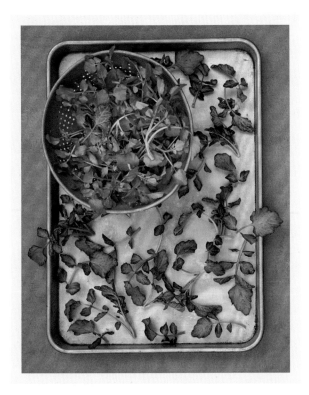

WILD WATERCRESS

Wild watercress has dark green pointed or round leaves and tough, woody stems. It is more pungent than cultivated watercress, especially when the sprigs have tiny white flowers. It truly grows in water. You can even forage it from streams. If you do, be sure the water around wild watercress is not polluted. Even clear water can contain bacteria, so check with someone who has local knowledge.

OTHER CRESSES

Tiny mustard cress sprouts and upland cress with large round leaves are not directly related to watercress.

Conventionally grown watercress is sprayed with pesticide, so consider buying organic. Hydroponic watercress, grown in hothouses, is not sprayed.

Watercress should have dark green—or garnet red—leaves and upright, succulent stems. Avoid watercress that is wilted, yellowed, or has spotted or folded leaves. Also avoid watercress with flowers; it will be tough and very bitter. We used to find teeny tiny snails on watercress and an occasional ladybug. I sometimes find snails again lately and take them to mean the watercress is really fresh.

How to Buy and Store

Bunches should be buried in or displayed on crushed ice, or standing in a tray of water.

At Asian markets watercress may be well-priced. It sells briskly so it is always fresh.

Remember that the bottom one-third to one-half of the stems must be discarded, along with sprigs that have bruised stems or crushed leaves. After trimming, a 6-ounce bunch of watercress makes salad for 6 or a bed under 4 servings of chicken. A smaller bunch serves two.

Bagged watercress is ready to use and yields 6 packed cups, roughly the same as a large bunch. So a bag that costs twice as much as a bunch still makes sense because of the waste you avoid and the prep time you save.

Watercress is very perishable, so use the day you buy it or the next day.

At the store, I put each bunch into a large plastic bag, blow into the bag, and knot it closed, creating an air cushion that protects the watercress.

At home, promptly remove any banding and spread out the sprigs, discarding broken sprigs or ones with bruised, bent leaves. Store watercress in a container with an inch of water in the bottom. Set a folded paper towel on top of the watercress and drape a plastic bag loosely over the container. Set the container on the top shelf in the refrigerator. Alternatively, wrap a moist paper towel around the bottom of the stems, roll the bunch in a paper towel, and slip it into a resealable plastic bag. Seal the bag and store it in the crisper drawer in the refrigerator— as always, away from apples and other fruits that emit ethylene gas.

Basic Watercress Techniques

WASHING

Just before using, swish watercress sprigs in a large bowl of cold water, then spin or pat the watercress dry.

PREPPING

Plucking Chefs pluck the individual leaves off of watercress. The rest of us take either a Zen or an efficient way.

Pinching tender sprigs off the stalk is the Zen way. It yields the most cress. Consider it a meditation.

Lining up a handful of stalks and chopping 1 to 3 inches off the end is the quick way to separate the tough part from the tender sprigs. Some tough stems get through, but this is what I usually do.

COOKING

Direct heat toughens watercress. A short plunge into boiling water, about 3 seconds, before stir-frying or other cooking, avoids this. The watercress should just turn vivid green and be slightly limp. Alternatively, removing from the heat, stir raw watercress into hot soup or risotto just before serving it, or arrange it as a bed under hot food like chicken cutlets and let the heat wilt it.

Five Ways to Use Watercress

Combine with potato and leek for a creamy soup

·

Wrap into a nori handroll with brown rice and carrots

·

Add a shot of watercress juice to chilled tomato juice

·

Stir-fry with ginger and garlic

·

Drizzle watercress, endive, and grapefruit sections
with mustard-grapefruit vinaigrette

WATERCRESS RECIPES

WATERCRESS DEVILED EGGS

CHILLED WATERCRESS SOUP

ASPARAGUS, WATERCRESS, AND RADISH SALAD WITH BITTERS VINAIGRETTE

SPICY CHOPPED SALAD

ENDIVE, WATERCRESS, AND PEAR SALAD

POTATO SALAD WITH GREEN PEAS AND WATERCRESS

BANGKOK BEEF SALAD

AVOCADO AND WATERCRESS TARTINE

SMOKED SALMON, GOAT CHEESE, AND WATERCRESS WRAP

WATERCRESS TACOS WITH QUESO FRESCO

GLORIOUS GREEN JUICE

ACKNOWLEDGMENTS

WRITING A COOKBOOK IS A VOYAGE. LIKE ALL JOURNEYS, IT requires curiosity, perseverance, collaboration, and serendipity. Traveling from vision to words, from soil and farms to my kitchen and now to yours, has involved digging, discoveries, and unexpected delights. These people helped along on this journey to making this a beautiful, delicious work with substance.

For providing information and for the greens to use, even when they were out of season, thank you Ron Binaghi, Jr., at Stokes Farm, Rick Bishop at Sweet Mountain Berry Farm, Nevia No and Bodhitree Farm, Georgeann Brennan and lavierustic.com, B&W Quality Growers, Tom Nunes and Matt Seeley at Foxy, everyone at Frieda's Finest, Margaret Hoffman at GrowNYC, David Karp, Barbara Sibley at La Palapa, Robert Schuller at Melissa's Produce, the Miglorelli family, Paffenroth Farms, Paulette Satur at Satur Farms, my local purveyors Agata & Valentina, A Matter of Health, and Whole Foods Markets. To Alice Bender and Dori Mitchell at the American Institute for Cancer Research, and to Ashley Koff, R.D., special thanks.

For your indispensible work and culinary skills in testing recipes and problem solving, Katie Wittenberg (and Meryl Rososfsky for connecting us), Brooke Jackson, and Lani Bloom. Doubly to Lani for carefully turning my indecipherable drafts into clear, consistent recipes and chapters.

To my brain trust, culinary and otherwise, thank you for inspiration, perspective, and invaluable information: Elizabeth Andoh, Cara DeSilva, Sari Gluckin, Hilary Maler, Rick Rogers, Marie

Simmons, Akasha Richmond, and Amrit Richmond. And to Charles Salzberg and fellow writers at the Writer's Voice, despite despising kale! Also Joan Emery, and my much-missed godmother, Muriel Sholin Miller.

A cookbook needs meticulous editing and the right physical expression for its content. Thank you, Pamela Cannon, Betsy Wilson, Shona McCarthy, Ellen Scordato (copy editor), Melanie Gold and Marie Thompson (proofreaders), and Anna Bauer (art director). Plus Catherine Adams at Inkslinger. And to rock star photographer Ben Fink, food stylist Lori Powell with Tara Clark, Joe Tully, et al., for the incomparable photographs.

Creating a cookbook requires lots of eating. To sharing and enjoying, thank you, Marianne Meischeid, Marsha Weiner, Amand Bosca, Sydney Fox, Ruth and Liam Flaherty, the Bernsteins, Amrit, and the staff at 460.

Heartfelt thanks to friends and colleagues who kept me sane through deadlines and frustrations, especially Akasha, Barney, Brenda, Elizabeth, Esther, Joan, Marianne, Sydney, and Wai.

To Wendy Sherman, my super agent, who shares a love of kale and who made this happen. Thank you for being there every step of the way.

Deepest apologies to anyone I have missed.

INDEX

DANA JACOBI is the author or co-author of fifteen cookbooks, including the bestselling *12 Best Foods Cookbook* and *Cook & Freeze: 150 Delicious Dishes to Serve Now and Later*. Two of them were nominated for the James Beard Foundation Book Award. She writes "Something Different," a bi-weekly column for The American Institute for Cancer Research and has written for *Cooking Light, Food & Wine,* and *The New York Times*. An early adapter of digital media, she posted Dana's Market Basket at Prevention.com. As Food & Wine editor for Prodigy, one of the first digital media sites, she posted The Bytable Feast, one of the first food blogs, from 1988 to 1993. Along with teaching cooking and developing recipes, she now blogs at danadish.tumblr.com. Dana lives in New York City. When not cooking, she is knitting.

danajacobi.com

Instagram.com/danajacobi

danadish.tumblr.com